THE
POISON PATH
HERBAL

"Coby Michael's *The Poison Path Herbal* is THE book that witches on the Poison Path have long been waiting for. It is an intense ride through the history and folklore of baneful plants, with exceedingly clear instructions on how to not only successfully grow them in your own garden but it also thoroughly details their proper preparation and usage on both magical and mundane levels. This is truly an important addition to the library of any apothecary or hedge rider."

TARA-LOVE MAGUIRE, COAUTHOR
OF *BESOM, STANG, AND SWORD*

"Reading *The Poison Path Herbal* is like sitting around a fire on a moonlit midsummer night conversing with a master of occult secrets. Brilliantly discussing Renaissance magic and herbalism; Greek, Roman, Egyptian, and Norse mythology; Biblical lore; and modern understandings of plant medicines; Michael seamlessly laces botanical science with entheogenic enchantment throughout this engaging work. In the process he outlines the Poison Path, showing the various mysteries and divine associations of Venus, Saturn, and Mercury. Read closely and carefully, as this book is not for the faint of heart. Michael is a *real* witch, and this is a book of *real* witchcraft, which includes recipes to make your own psychoactive tinctures, incense, beer, tea, and ointments. Hell—he even teaches you how to grow the magical plants yourself! The Psychedelic Renaissance has been waiting for a book like this—an *advanced* entheogenic grimoire for the witchy, the wyld, and the wyrd."

THOMAS HATSIS, AUTHOR
OF *THE WITCHES' OINTMENT*

"Coby exquisitely, with much research and deep respect, presents venefic, malefic, cthonic, and pure Poison Path magic, ethnobotany, and history at its finest. This is an essential book for any serious poisoner and herbalist."

JACLYN CHERIE, OWNER
OF THE NEPHILIM RISING

"Coby beautifully combines history, folklore, science, and magic in *The Poison Path Herbal* with a compelling and charismatic writing style, drawing on years of practice and experience. It is an informative and poetic resource—a powerful introduction to the Poison Path, and a reference for more advanced students."

IAN VERTEL, FOUNDER AND
OWNER OF POISON PLANT CULT

THE
POISON PATH
HERBAL

Baneful Herbs,
Medicinal Nightshades,
and
Ritual
Entheogens

COBY MICHAEL

Park Street Press
Rochester, Vermont

Park Street Press
One Park Street
Rochester, Vermont 05767
www.ParkStPress.com

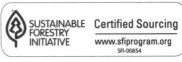

Text stock is SFI certified

Park Street Press is a division of Inner Traditions International

Cataloging-in-Publication Data for this title is available from the Library of Congress

ISBN 978-1-64411-334-9 (print)
ISBN 978-1-64411-335-6 (ebook)

Printed and bound in the United States by Lake Book Manufacturing, Inc.
The text stock is SFI certified. The Sustainable Forestry Initiative® program
promotes sustainable forest management.

10 9 8 7 6 5 4

Text design and layout by Virginia Scott Bowman
This book was typeset in Garamond Premier Pro and Gill Sans with Subversia and
Harman used as display typefaces

To send correspondence to the author of this book, mail a first-class letter to the
author c/o Inner Traditions • Bear & Company, One Park Street, Rochester, VT
05767, and we will forward the communication, or contact the author directly at
www.thepoisonersapothecary.com.

To my grandparents,
for showing me the beauty and magic
of the natural world

Danger! Toxic!
. . . .
Many of the plants discussed within this
book are poisonous. If used improperly, they
can cause illness and even death. It is important when
working with baneful herbs that you take extra precautions,
such as wearing gloves and protective eye coverings, using tools
designated for poisonous plants, and clearly labeling any dangerous
formulas to protect yourself and others. The information in this book
can be dangerous in the wrong hands! Please do not use this information
to poison an unsuspecting partner or launch any other diabolical schemes.
All of the details in this book are for informational purposes only and are
not meant to diagnose, prescribe treatment, or go against the advice of
your physician. When implementing any of the information or techniques
described here, you are doing so at your own risk. Consult with your
physician before experimenting with new plants, especially if you
are taking any medication, and avoid them if you have a heart
condition or are pregnant. There are many safe and powerful
ways to work with these plants without consuming them.
Neither the author nor the publisher is responsible
for any adverse effects that come from
using the information in this
book.

Contents

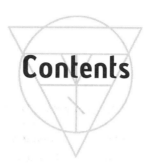

—————✷—————

PART 3
THE POISON PATH IN PRACTICE

Introduction

$\mathcal{T}$he Poison Path, as it has become known, is a branch of occult herbalism combined with entheogenic ritual practice, phyto-chemistry, and magic. The Poison Path is not limited to traditions of witchcraft or paganism. Although it is inherently animistic, there are no dogmas or institutions that restrict the use of this knowledge.

The Poison Path Herbal is focused on the magical and spiritual uses of baneful herbs, entheogens, and plant spirit allies, as well as their history and mythology. I personally came to know the uses of these plants through the practice of witchcraft and folk herbalism. It is through this lens that I have gained my own personal gnosis in regard to the intimate connections that some of these plants share with the practice of witch-craft and the ancient cultures that preceded Christianity.

Baneful refers to the ability of a thing to cause harm, and because of this threat, the baneful thing becomes taboo and gains a sinister repu-tation. In this case, we are talking about baneful herbs: herbs capable of causing bodily harm and sometimes death. They are plants that have been used for murder, execution, magic, and medicine through-out human history. Their prominent and often maligned place in the human pharmacopoeia is owing to their potency. Baneful herbs make powerful medicines and are often valued for their pain-relieving and sleep-inducing properties. Many of the plants in this category have a profound effect on human perception.

Entheogens are substances with the ability to generate spiritual expe-riences and altered consciousness within an individual or group. As with any mind-altering substance, the atmosphere and intention are a major influence on the experience. Entheogens are known for their ability to open us up to the spirit world through altering consciousness in order to work magic, prophesy, and commune with spirits. Through ritual and reverence, we are able to access the entheogenic effects of these plants. By changing human perception in subtle or extreme ways, they give us access to the divine, the otherworldly, and the arcane. While there are many substances that make up the entheogenic pharmacopoeia, they are not always used for spiritual purposes. Some substances, such as cocaine, tobacco, and caffeine, are predominantly consumed for recreational use. However, their entheogenic applications are not without merit.

Many entheogenic plants, such as belladonna, poppy, and datura, are also known for their baneful nature. They are powerful botanicals that if taken improperly could cause death. In addition to their poisonous properties, baneful herbs have a naturally dark and dangerous quality about them. Plants with thorns, carnivorous plants, and plants that grow around places we associate with the dead are all known for their baneful or baleful natures. Baneful herbs with entheogenic properties are also powerfully medicinal when one has the knowledge of how to use them. They have been used for centuries by virtually every human civilization for their medicinal and spiritual properties.

The Poison Path is a spiritually based practice that explores the esoteric properties of potentially deadly plants, and while many of them have entheogenic qualities, it was their poisonous nature that first attracted me. While the study of ritual entheogens can keep one busy for decades, we should not assume that they are the only way of accessing certain states of consciousness. It is a subcategory or supplemental set of tools and knowledge that can be utilized to enhance one's spiritual tradition. Many techniques exist for entering trance, altering perceptions, and encouraging spiritual experiences that do not require the use of mind-altering substances. These plants are not deities, and an entire tradition is not built up around them. The plants that belong to the Poison Path are among many guides and allies that we will meet along the way. Their entheogenic properties are the physical manifestation of the teaching powers that the spirits of these plants possess. Each plant spirit has an individual and complex personality.

I came to work with these plant spirit allies years ago through my study of traditional witchcraft, folk herbalism, and the animistic traditions of pre-Christian Europe. My research in modern witchcraft practices would sometimes offer a mention of one of the Old World witching herbs but seldom any serious or useful information. Knowledge of these powerful plants seems to have been kept out of modern witchcraft and its plant lore for some time, only recently making its way back. I think that knowledge of these plants has been kept secret or omitted from the wider magical community out of a desire to be more socially acceptable and distance the community from the drug culture of the 1960s and '70s. Instead of working with plant spirit allies, altered states of consciousness were achieved through meditation, chanting, and other shamanic techniques.

As one becomes intimate with the characteristics of these plants, shared traits become noticeable. Many of the hexing herbs of European witchcraft derive from the Solanaceae, or nightshade family. They are surrounded by superstition and lore, initially appearing to be fantastical, like the secret names for more mundane ingredients like bat's wing or eye of newt. Upon further investigation, similar themes in mythology begin to emerge. Many of these plants are mythically associated with deities and spirits of the underworld, the night, and magic—for example, Hecate, Circe, and Medea, who are renowned for their knowledge of poisons, potions, and witchcraft.

The plants are connected to deities of magic and witchcraft, ancient spirits credited with bringing knowledge to humanity. Many ancient cultures have similar myths about renegade gods coming to Earth to gift humanity with some sort of knowledge. Spirits from the wilderness or the underworld emerge at times to school an individual in the arcane arts. Each myth seems to contain a seed of an earlier source, allowing us to trace the origins of the ideas surrounding these important botanicals far back in human history. Among the stories and lore surrounding these plants are planetary and elemental correspondences attributed to them. These stories and associations give us clues to the nature of the spirits that dwell within and around these plants. Their innate energies can be honed by the magical practitioner to bring about a desired effect. Once an intimate understanding of their nature is formed, we can delve deeper into our own personal gnosis surrounding these plant spirit allies. Throughout this book, we will look at the mythological origins of many of these herbs, their legends, and the superstitions that have formed around them. Through an investigation of their esoteric associations, we can learn how to communicate with the genius of the plant and add powerful symbolic nuance to our rituals.

Medieval superstition has connected many of these plants with the Christian devil and with evil spirits in general, and a culture of fear and trepidation was encouraged around them. It has been suggested that some of the accounts of witchcraft during this period resulted from hallucinations brought on by their consumption. One thing is for certain: the connection that these plants have with magic, the spirit world, and the beings that have brought knowledge of such things to humanity is undeniable. These plants have an innate affinity with the nocturnal world of spirit and the arcane secrets hidden in the earth.

Not every plant in this category is a deadly toxin or a mind-expanding psychedelic. Some are aphrodisiacs or stimulants that may be used for ecstatic ritual celebration. Others are sedatives or hypnotics that can be employed for prophetic dreaming or divination, and still others allow us to travel beyond our bodies or summon spirits to our circle. They serve as catalysts of the *ars magica,* the magical arts, acting as teachers and familiars. These plants have a predisposition to the occult arts of a witch's private practice and can teach us more about ourselves and the many worlds out there.

This book seeks to provide information to people who would like to work with these plants in a spiritual or magical context. It is a compendium of history, lore, and scientific information along with some of my own personal insights and discoveries. The book is divided into three parts. Part 1 is an introduction to the Poison Path. It takes a look at the history of poison plants and how they have been used for medicine, murder, and magic since ancient times. The Poison Path is a nebulous practice, and to better define it there are explanations of important terminology and key concepts in this part. The connection between baneful herbs and witchcraft is explored here, along with the topic of using plant entheogens in magical practice. This section concludes with a chapter on the infamous witches' flying ointment, allegedly used by witches in the Middle Ages to fly to their sabbat meetings. Flying ointments are a popular tool for Poison Path practitioners, and this chapter discusses not only their history but also how to make them.

Part 2 is part herbal compendium, part grimoire. This section outlines some of the more esoteric concepts associated with poison plant magic. It contains a detailed description of each plant and its magical correspondences. Each monograph provides insight into the characteristics of the individual plant spirit through a telling of the myths and lore connecting these plants to the world of magic. This part is divided into three main categories based on the three energetic currents represented by the celestial bodies Saturn, Mercury, and Venus. While the overall theme of this book is Saturnian, since Saturn rules all poisonous plants, there are other qualities that manifest themselves as well. These are concepts and energies that are quintessential to the witch's practice and define what we do as witchcraft. The three often overlapping currents, or energetic themes, are reflected in the repertoire of the classical witch archetype. They are central to witch lore, reflected in the deities and spirits most intimately connected to the legacy of witchcraft. It is through these currents that I endeavor to establish a better understanding of the plants included in this book. We explore this threefold categorization using examples from astrology, alchemy, and occult symbolism. We examine each plant's magical correspondences, ritual uses, medicinal applications, and chemistry. You will be introduced to various deities and spirits that align with the chapter's theme along with recipes and magical operations that are either Saturnian, Mercurian, or Venusian.

Saturn is presented first. He can be considered the witch father, the horned god. Workings associated with Saturn are dark in nature, including spirit descent, maleficia, working with chthonic spirits, and necromancy. Venus, presented second, is the witch queen. She can be seen in all of the powerful goddess archetypes and also rules the arts of herb craft.

Venus can be found in workings of glamour magic,* manipulation and coercion, sex magic, and aphrodisia. In our cosmology Mercury can be thought of as the divine child. He is the immortal progeny of the divine parents, a light-bearing figure, a traveler and shape-shifter. Mercury is one of the most important figures to magical practitioners, manifesting in many forms. Otherworld travel, spirit communication, shape-shifting, divination, and alchemy are within the realm of Mercury. By studying the nuances in the information that we have available about these plants, we can associate them with one or more of these categories.

"The Poison Path in Practice" is the title of part 3. A big part of the Poison Path is about working with these plants in physical ways to receive nonphysical effects. Since many of the botanicals are very potent and potentially dangerous, practitioners must have a deep understanding of the plants they are working with. This section provides a strong foundation on which to begin creating your own herbal formulations. There is more information in this section on what entheogens are and how they can benefit one's spiritual practice. In addition to instructions on preparation and formulation, there is also information on the various extraction processes that can be used and which ones are most effective. There are many recipes in chapter 9 that provide examples of the use of poisonous plants in both medicine and magic. While some of the recipes come from historical sources, many are my own personal formulations. Chapter 10 details how to grow each plant from seed, including tips on germination and care of the plant through to harvesting and drying. Many green practitioners want to be involved in every step of the process. This is a powerful way to really connect with the plant spirit and receive its medicine.

By providing a wealth of ideas and practices as well as useful and accurate information to draw from, I aim to encourage you to embark on your own exploration with these powerful plant spirit allies.

---

*Glamour magic is the magic of casting illusions and creating auras so that people see what you want them to see. Glamours can be cast over people, places, and things. The effect of the glamour depends on its intention.

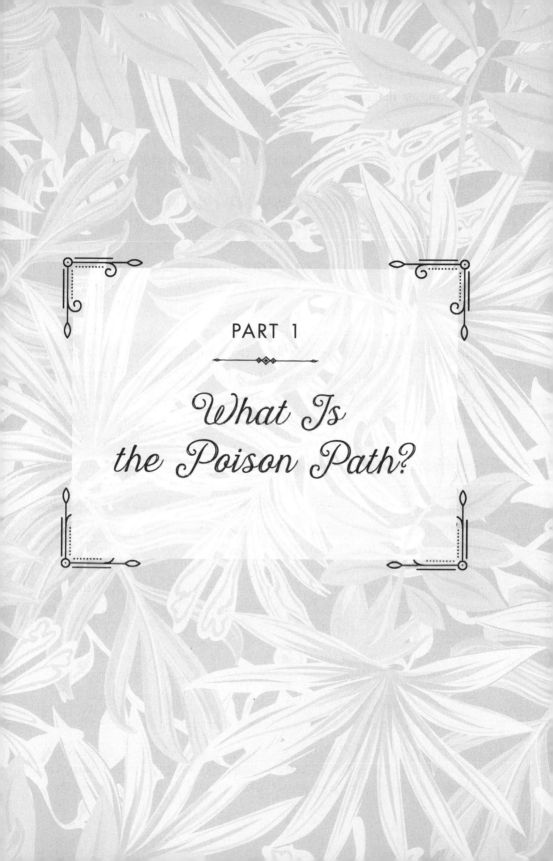

PART 1

What Is
the Poison Path?

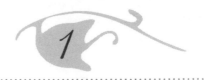

Basic Knowledge for the Poison Path

Entheology, Ethnobotany, and the Solanaceae

To tread the Poison Path requires drawing on knowledge from several areas: chemistry, alchemy, herbalism, folklore, and history. It also incorporates ethnobotany and entheology, fields of study that encompass many different cultures and time periods and are not limited to a specific tradition or a single group of plants.

Key to the path is becoming familiar with the Solanaceae or nightshade family of plants and their alkaloids. Since many of these plants can be dangerous in a variety of different ways, it is important to know a little bit about their chemistry and their action on human physiology.

SOLANACEAE IN THE GARDEN OF SHADOW

There are no plants more specifically associated with witchcraft and the devil than those that belong to the family of nightshade, the Solanaceae. *Solanaceae* means "to soothe," and these plants are valued for their pain-relieving and sedative properties. This category consists of the infamous plants of the medieval witch's garden, all of them feared and revered for their healing powers and their ability to loosen the shackles of the physical body, thereby freeing the spirit. In legend these plants were in the garden of Hecate, queen of the witches, who possessed knowledge of the uses for all the baneful herbs. She passed her knowledge on to her daughter Circe and the witch Medea, both of whom were well-known *pharmakeus,* an ancient term for a person knowledgeable about the medicinal and magical properties of plants.

The hexing herbs of the Solanaceae family—deadly nightshade, datura, mandrake, and henbane—share similar effects due to their chemistry, according to pharmacologist Louis Lewin. They have the property of calling forth "disorders of the brain, including peculiar excitation followed by depression."

We find these plants associated with incomprehensible acts on the part of the fanatics, raging with the flames of frenzy and fury and persecuting not only witches and sorcerers but mankind as a whole. Garbed in the cowl, the judge's robe, and the physician's gown, superstitious folly instituted diabolical proceedings in a trial of the devil and hurled victims into the flames or drowned in blood. Magic ointments or witches' philters procured for some reason and applied with or without intention produced effects which the subjects themselves believed in, even stating that they had intercourse with evil spirits, had been on the Brocken and danced at the Sabbat with their lovers, or caused damages to others by witchcraft. (Lewin 1998, 190)

Within the Solanaceae family are several plants that go by the name *nightshade.* They are all relatives of this larger category with their own distinct attributes. Some of the more common varieties that grow abundantly in Europe and North America, in addition to deadly nightshade (*Atropa belladonna*), are black nightshade (*Solanum nigrum*) and woody nightshade (*Solanum dulcamara*). These plants are also related to vegetables like pepper, tomato, and potato, which display similar characteristics, most evident in the shape of their flowers, which have five petals and sepals. Some flowers are bell or trumpet shaped, while others resemble stars. The berries range in color depending on the variety of the plant. The berries of black nightshade and deadly night-shade are black or deep purple. The berries of bittersweet nightshade start out green and, like a ripening tomato, go from yellow to orange and finally red.

In addition to the common varieties, there are those that are rarer, comprising the three thousand different species of this diverse family. Other plants like hemlock and wolfsbane are also known for their supernatural associations and are connected to witches and their patron spirits, capable of enhancing magical acts in their own unique ways. Many of these plants gained their arcane reputations through their poisonous nature, which connected them to infernal deities and, in later medieval lore, to the practice of witchcraft. In antiquity, sorcery was a common practice sought out by anyone in need of otherworldly assistance; however, there was a division between the practice of sorcery and black magic. This type of magic contrasted with the socially acceptable propitiation of the gods.

Astrologically, the nightshades are under the dominion of Saturn, known as the greater malefic, ruler of all poisonous plants and creatures. Many plants also have secondary planetary and elemental correspondences that further influence how they interact with our magic. For example, although the nightshades are Saturnian, they also have connections to Venus and Mercury. Other poisonous plants are connected by lore to Jupiter, Uranus, and Neptune and are used for their visionary, consciousness-expanding capabilities.

Many more practitioners are opening up to the idea of exploring these plants as spiritual allies in magical practice despite their reputation for being too dangerous to work with. However, as we integrate these chthonic and Saturnian energies that are a prominent part of traditional craft practices, we learn to work with our own shadow as well as the darker forces of the natural world. Much importance and inquiry has been placed on specific dosage and how to prepare formulas for entheogenic use through ingestion. Although there is a growing body of information based on experimental practices from modern practitioners, and some obscure medical references for the use of these plants, this is where one is largely left to walk the Poison Path for one-self. While there are guidelines and more information available with an increasing number of practitioners sharing their entheogenic experiences, personal exploration and learning are key.

There are several ways to work with these powerful spirits, just as there are for those plants used for healing. By using flower essences, ritual incense, oils, fetishes, and charms, one can come to understand safer esoteric ways of working with baneful herbs. The hallucinogenic and trance-inducing properties that they have are a small facet of the rich spiritual properties that can come from a working partnership with these botanical allies.

The variations in alkalinity among different plants and the many factors that contribute to how concentrated the alkaloids are in any given plant are part of the unpredictability characteristic of these teaching plants of a darker nature. They are the tricksters and shape-shifters of the plant world. They can act as both poison and panacea and teach us about boundaries and limitations that we would otherwise not approach. Their visions are often terrifying; their amnesiac qualities can sneak up on a practitioner who may not realize he or she was delirious until the effects of the plant have begun to subside.

ALKALOIDS

Possibly one of the most important words to the study of entheogens on the Poison Path is *alkaloid*. Alkaloids are the active chemicals within the plants that allow them to do what they do. They are responsible for all the effects the plants have on our brain chemistry and are also the medicinal components of the plants. Many plants contain alkaloids, but it is not immediately apparent what purpose these chemicals serve for the plants themselves. It is likely that these powerful chemicals are simply by-products of their chemical processes. The fact that they serve little purpose for the plants but have such profound effects on humans is a testament to nature's grand design. In this way, these plants are truly of the gods.

Alkaloids are compounds with a complex organic structure and occur naturally in plants, fungi, and animals. They contain carbon, oxygen, hydrogen, and nitrogen and are categorized based on their specific structure (Schultes 1976, 16). There are thousands of alkaloids that belong to different categories. Twenty-five thousand alkaloids are derived from plants. They have diverse and important physiological effects on humans and other mammals. Alkaloids are categorized based on their chemical structure, having a common heterocyclic nucleus such as indole, pyrrolizidine, and tropane.

The term *alkaloid* was developed in 1818 by K. F. W. Meissner (1792–1853), a German pharmacist. The names of specific alkaloids are based on their natural origin, using the name of a prototypal alkaloid group of the plant family (Funayama and Cordell 2015, 2–6). Morphine, strychnine, hyoscyamine, ephedrine, and nicotine are all alkaloids that have had an impact on humanity. Hallucinogenic alkaloids are indole alkaloids such as ergoline used in the synthesis of LSD, ibogaine from a hallucinogenic shrub in Africa, and harmaline found in Syrian rue (Schultes 1976, 43). Other alkaloids are more mildly hallucinogenic, acting differently on the body. These pseudohallucinogens or deliriants, such as the tropane alkaloids, are more dangerous at hallucinogenic doses.

Covering all the different plant-based alkaloids is beyond the scope of this book and my expertise. There are some comprehensive academic texts out there that cover the topic of alkaloids thoroughly, and I have included them in the works cited at the end of the book. The focus of this book is to explore the plants containing the tropane alkaloids, the Solanaceae family. The Solanaceae, or nightshades, comprise a group of plants historically associated with magic and witchcraft. The plants within this group have a long history of ritual use and are associated with spirits allied to the arcane arts. They have been used as funerary herbs, offerings to deities, and ingredients in spells and as a means of opening a doorway to the spirit world. While the Solanaceae are the crux of this book, I also explore other plants that are prominent in folklore and pagan myth.

Tropane Alkaloids

Tropane alkaloids, which are found in the nightshade family, are characterized by their unique nitrogen bridge or tropane ring. The tropane alkaloids are secondary metabolites, which means that the plant's survival is not contingent on their presence. These naturally occurring nitrogen compounds are basic, having an alkaline pH.

Some of the most commonly discussed solanaceous alkaloids are atropine, hyoscyamine, hyoscine or scopolamine, and solanine. These chemicals are found in plants like deadly nightshade, mandrake, henbane, and thorn apple. They are present in different amounts and combinations depending on the plant, and each alkaloid has a slightly different effect.

Atropine (dl-hyoscyamine) was isolated in the 1830s and was a cornerstone in the study of neurochemistry. It led to the discovery of the neurotransmitter acetylcholine (Datta and Rita 2011). The half-life of atropine is four hours, meaning it takes the body four hours to metabolize half the amount of atropine ingested. However, symptoms may last twenty-four to forty-eight hours due to decreased gastrointestinal motility (digestion). Atropine is easily absorbed by the gastrointestinal tissues and mucous membranes but does not penetrate the skin as effectively.

Hyoscyamine is found in fresh plant material and is a depressant. It racemizes (converts) to atropine (dl-hyoscyamine) in dry plant material and/or in liquid extraction. Atropine is a stimulant and at low doses (0.5–1 mg) leads to mild excitation, while 10 mg of atropine results in the central depression of life functions (Börsch-Haubold 2007).

Scopolamine (d-hyoscine) is responsible for fatigue, drowsiness, dreamless sleep, euphoria, and amnesia. At higher doses, it causes restlessness and hallucinations. Scopolamine is one of the alkaloids of the Solanaceae family. It is like atropine, an antagonist of the muscarinic cholinergic receptors (anticholinergics). Scopolamine is a hypnotic, having a shorter duration of effect on the peripheral nervous system than atropine. It can depress the central nervous system in a little as 0.5 mg (Alizadeh et al. 2014, 300).

Scopolamine is used today in medication for motion sickness and is generally applied in the form of a patch. It is also used topically for pain relief and is an effective analgesic. Scopolamine is easily absorbed by the skin, unlike atropine and hyoscyamine. Oftentimes these patches are worn by tourists traveling abroad, leading to increased intoxication and amnesia when consumed with alcohol. Scopolamine powder has been used by unscrupulous individuals as a means of committing numerous crimes. Scopolamine poisoning allegedly results in a "zombie-like" state, during which the victim is easily manipulated. Afterward, the poison causes amnesia, leaving no memory of the previous events. These qualities make scopolamine a dangerous tool for thieves and predators of all kinds.

Solanine is an allelochemical that occurs in some plants as a defense mechanism against competitive encroachment. Allelochemicals are released into the soil and interfere with the biomembranes of other plants, leading to death. Solanine, a glycoalkaloid present in black nightshade, woody nightshade, and other common Solanaceae, is also present in the leaves and stem of the potato plant. It can cause nausea, vomiting, dry mouth, abdominal pain, mydriasis, and seizures.

The tropane alkaloids act on the brain in unique ways. They are capable of activating the pineal gland, which corresponds to our third eye. The pineal gland senses changes between light and darkness even though it is deep inside the brain. By stimulating melatonin, these alkaloids can induce a dreamlike waking state. It is a state akin to lucid dreaming, which is further enhanced by darkness and ecstatic techniques.

The tropane alkaloids are *anticholinergic*. Anticholinergics are a group of substances that block the neurotransmitter acetylcholine in the central and peripheral nervous system. There are three types of anticholinergics; the tropane alkaloids are *antimuscarinic*, the most common of the three types. Acetylcholine is the chief neurotransmitter of the parasympathetic nervous system and activates muscarinic receptors in nerve cells, which contract smooth muscles. Atropine and scopolamine chemically resemble acetylcholine. They bind to the receptors but fail to stimulate the cell (antagonists), and thus nerve transmission is blocked. Blocking acetylcholine inhibits nerve impulses that affect the functioning of involuntary smooth muscles in the gastrointestinal tract, urinary tract, and lungs. This causes many of the symptoms for which tropane alkaloids are known.

Poisoning from these plants results in acute anticholinergic syndrome or toxidrome. Symptoms of tropane alkaloid poisoning are remembered with this common mnemonic: "Blind as a bat, mad as a hatter, red as a beet, hot as a hare, dry as bone, the bowel and bladder lose their tone, and the heart runs alone." Recreational users consider these plants the least enjoyable because of their side effects. They are commonly referred to as deliriants. Long-term use may result in physical and mental decline.

The effects of tropane alkaloids on the peripheral nervous system receptors on exocrine glands can cause poor coordination, decreased mucus production, anhidrosis (no sweating), and increased body temperature. The muscles in the bladder and urinary tract are affected, resulting in urinary retention. The mydriatic effects of pupil dilation cause light sensitivity (photophobia) and cycloplegia (inability to focus close up).

The effects on the central nervous system resemble delirium and consist of confusion, disorientation, euphoria or dysphoria, memory problems, loss of concentration, and illogical thinking. As tertiary amines, which are absorbable by the central nervous system, they result in anticholinergic syndrome manifesting as psychosis. They can cause visual disturbances such as seeing warped and textured surfaces, dancing lines, and imaginary spiders or insects. In addition to other visual disturbances, auditory and sensory disturbances occur as well. These can include phantom smells of smoke, visions of lifelike objects and figures, and the sensation of nonphysical presences. This explains the use of these plants in visionary workings and in the communication with spirits. Daniel Schulke coined the term *chronophagoi* or *time-eaters* to describe the effects of tropane alkaloids because of the loss of time due to their amnesiac effects.

ENTHEOGENS

All of the plants within this category, no matter their chemical action or level of toxicity, are in some way considered *entheogens*. The term *entheogen* was coined to replace the socioculturally loaded term *psychedelic* from the 1960s. It comes from two Greek words: *éntheos*, which means "full of the god, inspired and possessed," and *genésthai*, which means "to come into being."

Entheology is the study of entheogens, or plants that generate the divine within. Its name was conceived by a group of influential ethnobotanists in 1979: Carl A. P. Ruck, Jeremy Bigwood, Danny Staples, Jonathan Ott, and R. Gordon Wasson (Ruck et al. 1979). Ethnobotanists study the traditions of different cultures and the way that they use plants medicinally, spiritually, and ritually, as well as their practical uses. Entheology can be thought of as a specific branch of ethnobotany.

Not all entheogens are psychedelic or hallucinogenic; they exhibit a broad spectrum of effects from the most subtle to the most intense. Stimulants, sedatives, deliriants; and aphrodisiacs all alter human brain chemistry and perception in different ways. These different states, when entered ritually, can aid the practitioner in achieving his or her desired results. Entheogens are any substances, typically plant or animal based, that are used as spiritual and sacramental tools (Tupper 2009). Louis Lewin (1850–1929) used the term *phantastica*, derived from *phantasia*, a Greek word meaning "imagination, appearance," to describe the many plants within this category. Lewin's book *Phantastica*, published in 1929, is credited with beginning ethnobotany.

As mentioned earlier, entheogens are not simply drugs. There are those spiritually oriented individuals who practice the use of traditional ritual entheogens for their consciousness-expanding effects. These practitioners often call themselves psychonauts and experiment with a wide variety of entheogens, hallucinogens, and psychedelics. Recreational users often have very different and uncomfortable experiences when using these plants just for a high. The ritual preparation and spiritual understanding are paramount to unlocking the potential of these powerful allies. "Consider the degree by which the potential of entheogens comes not only from their neurophysiological effects, but also from social practices, rituals into which their use has been traditionally incorporated" (Tupper 2009, 503).

Many of these plants contain deadly toxins, and their effects can be debilitating and detrimental to cognition. Regular long-term use by recreational users can result in permanent damage and death. "Ritual context, however, offers psychospiritual safeguards that make the potential of entheogenic plant teachers to enhance cognition an intriguing possibility" (Tupper 2009, 503). Traditional ritual entheogens, as the name implies, help us connect with the spiritual forces in nature. They help us bring the essence of the divine into ourselves and access our own divine connection to the rest of the universe. They do this by facilitating initiatory experiences that, though not always pleasant, can give us a new perspective and expand our consciousness. Many modern practitioners of different forms of witchcraft and neoshamanism have a desire to work with these traditional plants.

By entering a spiritual relationship with such plants, we gradually gain a deeper understanding of their uses and the proper way to work with them, coming to know them first at a distance until a more intimate relationship is reached. These plants act as gatekeepers to spiritual understanding, and it is often through a balanced synergy that such understanding is achieved. Plant spirits are often just as, if not more, willing to partner with humans in the pursuit of spiritual and occult knowledge than other spirits because of humanity's close relationship with them. Many practitioners have specific plants with which they have developed a familiar relationship, and through this bond their work is enhanced.

ETHNOBOTANY, ETHNOPHARMACOLOGY, PHARMACOGNOSY

The cultural folklore, traditional remedies, and spiritual uses of plants are all part of the study of *ethnobotany*. Practitioners of esoteric herbalism, plant magic, and alchemy are already involved in the study of ethnobotany. By understanding the myths, legends, medicinal properties, and physical characteristics of plants, we gain a deeper understanding of their occult characteristics. Every bit of lore provides an additional layer of symbolism that can be incorporated into one's magical practice.

Ethnopharmacology is the study of the traditional medicines of different groups of people. Folk cures, traditional Chinese medicine, and ayurveda are all examples of *materia medica* collected by a group of people over time. Many traditional cures work homeopathically or require the synergy of multiple plants to be effective. An understanding of energy and balance is often required in these culturally based practices. Some cures work by nonphysical means that are not completely understood, though their effectiveness is well known within the culture.

Pharmacognosy is the study of naturally derived medicines. Many of the plants within this pharmacopeia have medicinal properties. Some have resulted in important discoveries in modern medicine and are still used by the pharmaceutical industry. Understanding how to use these powerful natural medicines safely is one of the lessons these plants have to teach us. The old Paracelsian dictum is often repeated by those on the Poison Path: *dosis sola facit ut venenum non fit* (only the dose permits something not to be poisonous). This basic principle of toxicology teaches that anything can be toxic if the dose is high enough. On the other hand, substances that are apparently toxic can have beneficial properties when the appropriate dose is found.

TREADING THE POISON PATH IN MODERN WITCHCRAFT

Modern advances in phytochemistry and plant medicine have taken us to a place where we as practitioners can blend science with magic; however, advances in the chemical extraction of these substances for pharmaceutical use have created a dangerous tool in the wrong hands. These powerful alkaloids in their pure state have resulted in many negative experiences and sickness in those seeking recreational highs by exploiting these sacred herbs. Many people, upon hearing of their use in spirit work and witch's flight, view these plants as magical potions, nothing more than a pill that can be taken to gain its prescribed effect. But these sacred plants are not a shortcut to spiritual knowledge or magical power, just as they are not pleasant highs to be chased by the recreational drug user. From a magical perspective, these plants cannot simply be reduced to something profane and utilitarian.

The baneful plants are autonomous entities offering experiential gnosis; the path of exploring their mysteries must be treaded individually. These plants do not give up their mysteries easily. Just as with animal spirits, an intimate bond must be forged on a one-to-one basis, and in many cases, the spirit does the choosing. Ritual and relationship are the keys to working with these plants and unlocking their mysteries. The ritual process is just as vital a part of this practice as the active components of the plants themselves. They are tricksters and sometimes adversaries, their effects and potency always changing. Many people are concerned about dosages, knowing that these plants are poisonous. I, however, think it is good that there are no universally prescribed dosages; no one can say for certain what one plant will do for another person. The prospect of potential poisoning and unpleasant side effects keeps the dabblers at bay.

It is important that we do not forget what brought us to these plants to begin with. Their practical use and growing prominence in modern witchcraft continue the ancient tradition with these powerful botanical allies. The lore surrounding these plants continues to grow and transform as we gain new insight through direct communion with these plant spirits.

2

A Brief History of Baneful Herbs

Medicine, Politics, and Magic

The plants traditionally associated with witchcraft have been used in medicine, politics, and magic by diverse groups throughout history and have shared infamous reputations and prominent places in myth since antiquity. Poisonous plants have played a pivotal role in shaping human history. Since ancient times, early humans made use of the power of plant toxins, whether discovered by chance or experimentation. The powerful effects of these substances elevated them to a mythical status.

The ancient Egyptians recorded their use in the Ebers Papyrus, among the oldest surviving medical texts documenting ancient herbal knowledge dated to circa 1550 BCE. The Ebers Papyrus combines the use of magic and botanical medicine, providing incantations and rituals with some of the recipes. Opium poppy, cannabis, and belladonna are among the herbs prescribed and were used in topical applications or steeped in wine to relieve pain and bring sleep (Crystalinks 2009).

Historically, belladonna and henbane have been used in ointments and liniments applied topically for pain. Mandrake was combined with opium to create a powerful anesthetic used by medieval physicians. Datura, a relative of the European thorn apple, is used in South America and Central America to create an amnesiac effect, which was used during childbirth to dull the pain and cause the patient to forget her experience. Loss of time is a common effect attributed to the tropane alkaloids.

BANEFUL PLANTS AS ENTHEOGENS

The use of entheogens as plant allies is common to humanity and has been a source of healing and knowledge for millennia. Entheogens have been used by many cultures around the world and have an extensive history in religious ritual and magic.

The Talmud and other Jewish writings suggest the entheogenic effects of incense used in temple fumigations. According to the Bible, God said to Moses, "Take unto thee sweet spices, stacte and onycha, and galbanum; these sweet spices with pure frankincense: of each shall there be a like weight. And thou shalt make it a perfume, a confection after the art of the apothecary, salted together, pure and holy" (Exodus 30:34–35). The Talmud adds ingredients with entheogenic qualities like spikenard, cassia, and myrrh.

The plants themselves have been elevated to a divine status, their stories told throughout history in myth and legend. Ancient cultures recognized their usefulness as medicinal herbs, but they did not neglect the powerful spiritual properties of these plants. Oftentimes, entheogenic plants and fungi were thought to be gifts from the gods and were treated as holy sacraments. A healer or shaman did not just use a plant for its chemical properties but also called upon the spirit of the plant to serve a specific purpose.

In animistic societies, these plants were viewed as independent entities with unique spirits and were sometimes anthropomorphized. The mandrake is perhaps the most famous example of this. The root, which resembles the human body, was thought to contain a spirit that, when cared for in the proper manner, would work in favor of the person keeping it. These plant fetishes, called manikins, homunculi, or, in German, *alraune,* were often passed down within families, from one generation to another. These powerful roots were so coveted that charlatans would often substitute the more common white bryony root in northern Europe, passing it off for genuine mandrake.

Another example would be the keeping and feeding of roots such as angelica root (*Angelica archangelica*), masterwort root

(*Imperatoria ostruthium*), and High John the Conqueror root (*Ipomoea jalapa*). Although these roots do not resemble a human form, they are often treated in the same way. Life is breathed into the root, and its spirit is awakened through cleansing and anointing, reminiscent of a kind of baptism. The root is then regularly empowered—spoken to and fed various oils and powders—to strengthen the keeper's intentions. The root itself stands as a proxy for the powerful spirit that it contains.

POISONOUS BOTANICALS IN WARFARE AND POLITICS

The knowledge of botanical toxins was well established in the ancient world. Tribal communities and prehistoric hunter-gatherer societies used poison-tipped arrows to take down large game. The Atharva Veda, an ancient Sanskrit text, circa 900 BCE, mentions poisoning arrow heads with aconite (Bisset 1989, cited in Borgia 2019). They were eventually used in warfare against human enemies.

In Homer's *Iliad* and *Odyssey*, poisoned arrows were used in battle (Mayor 2009). The word *toxic* derives from the Greek *toxikón*, which gave us the Latin *toxicum*. The root of this word also connects to *toxon*, meaning "bow." The Greek word for the yew tree is *taxon*, and yew was often the preferred wood for constructing bows and arrows. The yew is also one of the most toxic plants in the Mediterranean. This etymology shows us the connection between poisonous substances and weapons. Aconite or wolfsbane was commonly employed as an arrow poison. The Latin word *acontizo* means "to hurl a javelin," and *aconite* or *aconitum* come from the same Greek root word, *akoniton* (Borgia 2019).

The Scythians were known for their knowledge of poisons and antidotes. They had their own special poison called *scythicon* that they used on arrows. The Celts of Gaul used a toxin known as *limeum* to poison their arrows, which according to Pliny the Elder was a preparation made from the juice of the hellebore.

Poisonous plants were readily available in the ancient world, and the ancient Greeks and Romans made laws governing their use, such as the Lex

Cornelia de Maiestate (81–80 BCE), which attempts to categorize plant poisons, drugs, and medicines. Assassination through poison derived from baneful plants was a common tactic, especially within the Roman Empire.

Political life was a major aspect of being a citizen of ancient Greece and Rome. Aristocratic families and those with senatorial positions met on a regular basis to discuss governmental concerns. Politicians fought for power using eloquence and logic, in stark contrast to the tribal warlords in the Roman province of Germania. Under the guise of civilized government, politicians found more subversive means of eliminating opponents. Members of the aristocracy attempting to advance their own positions would employ the help of a poisoner-assassin to eliminate those standing in their way. This was often achieved in close proximity under the pretense of trust. In 54 CE, Agrippina, mother of the emperor Nero, hired a woman named Locusta to assassinate Claudius I. Locusta, a notorious poisoner known as a *venefica,* allegedly poisoned him using aconite. The infamous poisoner Canidia, written about by the Roman poet Horace, was feared by her contemporaries and was known for using a poison consisting of hemlock and honey (Retief and Cilliers 2019). The nature of poisoning is secretive and discreet, often making use of deceiving illusions. The poisoner may have a close relationship to the victim, such as being a friend or family member.

Mithridatium

So great was the fear of being poisoned that rulers in antiquity went to extreme measures to protect themselves. It wasn't uncommon for a monarch to have a servant test his food for poison before eating it himself. Apothecaries could be employed to create antidotes and poisons. One ruler is known for the extreme measures that he took to protect himself from his predecessor's fate. Mithridates VI, king of Pontus from 120 to 63 BCE, was one of the Roman Republic's most formidable enemies. With such a big target on his back, Mithridates went to great ends to protect himself from assassination by poison.

Under the instruction of the *agari,* a group of Scythian shamans, Mithridates attempted to immunize himself by ingesting small amounts of various poisons on a regular basis. According to legend and history, this semimythical account was a success. This process became known as *mithridatism* and has been employed in other instances of immunization as well. This technique depends on how the body metabolizes certain toxins. It was a dangerous technique of immunization, and Mithridates spent many years and went through many convicted criminals testing his poisons and antidotes.

On the other end of the spectrum of poison and antidotes, there was a legendary cure-all that was known as *mithridatium,* named after the ancient monarch. This panacea was sought after from antiquity into the Middle Ages. The coveted compound under the name *theriaca andromachi* or Venice treacle was made primarily in Venice during the Middle Ages. This medicine was only available to those who could afford it because of the number of ingredients needed and the long amount of time it took to produce. It allegedly consisted of around sixty-five ingredients, and it would take months to gather and prepare the necessary components. The treacle would then need to be fermented for at least a year before being used. The famous French apothecary Moyse Charas (1619–1698) published the formula in 1669 to help put an end to the Venetian monopoly on the theriac.

The Gift of Death

Emperor Chandragupta Maurya, founder and emperor of the Mauryan dynasty in India, is known for his unique use of poison to create a special type of assassin. The *visha kanyas,* or "poison maidens," were young women specially prepared from a young age to become assassin seductresses. The group, first organized by Chandragupta, operated between 320 and 298 BCE and is mentioned in the *Arthashastra,* an ancient Indian Sanskrit treatise on statecraft. The women were allegedly given a specific diet and ingested small amounts of various poisons over time, which eventually rendered their bodily fluids toxic to normal individuals. According to legend, they were not simply administrators of poison through food and drink; they *were* the poison. Given to Chandragupta's enemies as gifts, these women used their sexual charms to lull victims into a false sense of safety. The poisonous maidens killed their victims through intercourse, but reputedly, they could also kill with one touch—their victims realizing too late what had been done to them. These women of folklore were likely based on real women who were sent in as assassins to poison royal enemies through food and drink.

It was a common practice in antiquity to give gifts of fabric or garments; exchanging garments as a way to bestow honor is an ancient theme. Throughout history, gifts of clothing are given to literally or figuratively confer authority, protection, and honor. To cover someone with a mantle is to bestow upon them the blessings symbolized therein.

However, mantles and garments can also confer danger and death. In mythology, Morgan le Fay gave King Arthur a mantle meant to immolate him, and the sorceress Medea in the Greek epic poem *Argonautica* gave the nymph Creusa a poisoned mantle meant to consume her in fire. The poisoning of garments is a peculiar practice based on traditions of gift giving: the poisoning is accomplished under a pretense of trust and safety. Foreign monarchs have unknowingly accepted these contaminated gifts out of decorum, to avoid insulting the gift giver. This real fear that garments carried disease led to strict taboos to ensure cleanliness and avoid contamination.

VENEFICIUM: POISON AND WITCHCRAFT

Concepts of contamination and contagion are part of many religious and spiritual practices. Traditions of taboo have developed around purification and cleanliness with both spiritual and physical components. The secretive nature of poisoning and its unseen effects on the body align it closely with classical ideas of witchcraft. Over the years, many have theorized that it is poison's secretive nature that has resulted in its long associations with harmful witchcraft. This real fear of the existence of poisoners and witches, often considered one and the same, resulted in outlawing practices of *maleficium or harmful witchcraft and veneficium or poisoning*. The poisoning of body and mind was sorcery to ancient societies. The plants that were used for their toxic and mind-altering qualities became associated with the witch's garden, a garden specifically designed to cultivate magical and medicinal plants that serve as allies of power and progress to those on the Poison Path.

3

The Witches' Flying Ointment

*O*intments were in widespread use as medicinal preparations long before their associations with witches and their sabbat meetings. Some of the earliest written recipes come from the *Trotula,* a collection of three twelfth-century Italian medical texts on women's health written in Salerno, Italy. The text is named for the historic figure Trotula of Salerno, a female physician credited with writing one of the texts. The *Trotula* texts circulated widely throughout medieval Europe.

These ointments were used to treat a wide variety of symptoms, and their creation was common knowledge. They were originally part of the pharmacopoeia of village herbalists and apothecaries. Ointments containing solanaceous and soporific (sleep-inducing) plants were common in premodern medicine. Many of them contained medicinal herbs that were known to have entheogenic properties. Their connection to diabolic witchcraft did not begin until the Middle Ages. The lines became blurred between medieval superstition and folklore, the deluded beliefs of the Inquisitors, and actual pagan practices of pre-Christian Europe.

The idea that individuals used entheogenic ointments as magical catalysts prior to this time period is unlikely. However, preexisting documentation and archaeological discovery support the use of entheogenic plants such as henbane, fly agaric, and mandrake for ritual purposes throughout the ancient world. The plants would have been burned as incense or ingested by drinking an infusion of the plant in water or alcohol.

The existence of a witches' ointment was primarily a subject of debate between prosecutors and defendants in the witch trials themselves. There were those who believed that witches' sabbats were real and that the ointment enabled a witch to fly to these gatherings, often attended by the devil. The ointments that witches used for this purpose contained noxious and deadly ingredients, which was considered evidence of their iniquity. At best, these ointments were used by the devil to create delusions of the senses and prey on the weakened minds of those who partook in them. At worst, they were nefarious preparations used by the devil's agents to bewitch the innocent, work maleficia, and transport themselves to the witches' sabbat.

The other argument was that the witches' sabbat was a delusion induced by the hallucinogenic ingredients in these ointments; thus, the witches' sabbat did not exist and the accused were not guilty of crimes of witchcraft. The idea that these experiences were fantasies and visions brought on by these dangerous plants was used by those intellectuals with a more humanistic view to argue the innocence of those accused of witchcraft since they didn't literally meet with the devil.

This debate fueled a body of lore surrounding the witches' ointment. The majority of writings regarding such an ointment come from inquisitorial texts and those written by learned men interested in the topic. The writings of Inquisitors and demonologists largely contributed to the lore of the witches' ointment, called *unguentum sabbati* or *unguentum lamiarum*. This served to demonize traditional pagan ritual herbs, as well as flush out natural healers and rural herbalists. Hildegard von Bingen, in *Physica*, demonized many of the plants associated with pre-Christian practices in her descriptions of them, among them belladonna and mandrake (Hildegard 1998, 75). The lore perpetuated by the church is the basis for the modern understanding of the witches' flying ointment. Within the deluded superstitions of the witch hunters are grains of truth regarding the use of entheogenic plants by pre-Christian people.

The earliest surviving documented mention of a person using a flying ointment to meet Satan is from the trial testimony of Matteucia di Francesco in 1428, according to the comprehensive book on the topic, *The Witches' Ointment* by Thomas Hatsis. Matteucia was tried in Rome and burned at the stake for her purported "diabolical congregation."

(Hatsis 2015, 205). In *The Book of Sacred Magic of Abramelin the Mage,* Abraham of Worms (1362–1458) recounts being given an ointment by an old woman that gave him the ability to fly. In another early reference to flying ointments, Johannes Hartlieb (1410–1468), in *The Book of All Forbidden Arts, Heresy, and Sorcery,* published in 1475, stated that these ointments were composed by *unholden* (witches) by collecting seven herbs on their respective day of the week.

Sunday: Borage (*Borago officinalis*)
Monday: Honesty (*Lunaria annua*)
Tuesday: Vervain (*Verbena officinalis*)
Wednesday: Spurge (*Mercurialis annua*)
Thursday: Vetch (*Anthyllis barba*)
Friday: Maidenhair fern (*Adianthum capillus-veneris*)

The seventh herb to be collected on Saturday is omitted, which is interesting, considering that Saturn rules this day. It is likely that the seventh ingredient was a nightshade or other baneful herb. Since all the other ingredients are nonpsychoactive, the last ingredient would likely have contained a hallucinogenic component (Hatsis 2015, 177).

Another early mention of an ointment in connection with witches was in *De subtilitate verum* (The Subtleties of Things) written by Girolamo Cardano (1501–1576) in 1550. Cardano's twenty-one volume work is the first publication where witches and their ointments appear together. In book 18, *De mirabilius* (On Marvels), he lists the ingredients of the flying ointment as "fat of children, juice of parsley, aconite, cinquefoil, nightshade, soot." He also outlines the ointment's effect on the psyche: "theatres, pleasure gardens, banquets, beautiful ornaments, and clothing, handsome young men, kings [and] magistrates, demons, ravens, prisons, desert wastes, and torments" (Cardano, cited in Hatsis 2015, 189). In 1545, Andrés Laguna (1499–1559), a Spanish physician, botanist, and pharmacologist, gives one of the most reliable records of a soporific ointment after testing it on a patient. He describes the ingredients as some of "the very coldest and soporific herbs" (Laguna 1554).

In his *Magiae Naturalis* (Natural Magic), Giambattista della Porta (ca. 1535–1615) notes that the witches "smear all parts of the body, first rubbing them to make them ruddy and warm and to rarify whatever had been condensed because of the cold. When the flesh is relaxed and the pores opened up, they add the fat (or oil that is substituted for it)— so that the power of the juices can penetrate further and become stronger and more active no doubt." Porta lists the following ingredients for a flying ointment: "wild celery [hemlock], fat of children, juice of parsley, aconite, cinquefoil, nightshade, soot." Another recipe in the same book offers the following: "water parsnip, common acorum [calamus], cinquefoil, bat's blood, nightshade" (Porta 1558, book 2, chap. 26).

Karl Kieswetter (1854–1895) mixed an ointment based on Porta's recipe and described dreaming of flying in spirals (Harner 1973, 139). Flying, shape-shifting, and encountering monstrous creatures and entities were common in descriptions of people's experiences with these ointments. These experiences can be attributed to the mind-altering effects and delirium produced by the effects of tropane alkaloids.

The following two recipes are from *The Discoverie of Witchcraft* by Reginald Scot (1538–1599), first published in 1584. Scot intended his book to be an exposé, challenging the belief in and existence of witchcraft in an effort to prevent the persecution of vulnerable people, often poor and aged women.

> The fat of yoong children, and seeth it with water in a brasen vessell, reserving the thickest of that which remaineth boiled in the bottome, which they laie up and keepe, untill occasion serveth to use it. They put hereunto *Eleoselinum* [*Apium graveolens*], *Aconitum* [wolfsbane], *Frondes populeas* [poplar buds] and Soote.
>
> *Sium* [water parsnip-hemlock], *acarum vulgare* [*Acorus calamus*], *pentaphyllon* [cinquefoil], the bloud of a flitter-mouse [bat's blood], *solanum somniferum* [*Atropa belladonna*], & *oleum*. (Scot 1886, chap. 8)

The plants mentioned in medieval flying ointment recipes raise questions about their effectiveness and whether these recipes were used for their alleged purpose. Many of the ingredients listed either do not have any entheogenic properties or are extremely toxic. Plants like poison hemlock and wolfsbane are often listed as ingredients, and both are extremely toxic and nonhallucinogenic. I would not rub the juice of either of these plants on my skin! Deadly nightshade is one of the only plants listed that does have hallucinogenic properties as a deliriant. It appears that the recipes that surfaced around the time of the witch craze act only as a scare tactic. These recipes all contain practically the same ingredients, including the most deadly plants in Europe along with bat's blood and the fat of unbaptized children—sounding more like the idea of a witch hunter than someone well versed in herbalism.

Plants like henbane, mandrake, and datura were rarely used until later. These would have been safer and more effective ingredients as opposed to hemlock and wolfsbane for use in a witches' ointment. Henbane figures extensively in the folklore of Germanic peoples, and mandrake's reputation was widespread before even reaching northern Europe because it was prized as a fertility and love charm. While datura didn't enter the pharmacopoeia of northwestern Europe until the sixteenth and seventeenth centuries, henbane would have been a definite option for those knowledgeable about entheogenic plants. The fact that these plants are not more prominent in medieval flying ointment recipes raises questions about their authenticity as a preparation actually used by people believing themselves to be witches to induce trance and practice witchcraft.

In the middle of the twentieth century, German folklorist Will Erich Peuckert (1895–1969) experimented with an effective dose of henbane, mandrake, and datura. During his experiment, he and two other individuals fell into a deep sleep for twenty-four hours. Interestingly, they all reported similar experiences during this time. Michael Harner quotes him in *Hallucinogens and Shamanism,* describing his visions of "wild rides, frenzied dancing and other weird adventures . . . connected to medieval orgies" (Harner 1973, 139). Peuckert was subjected to ridicule for mentioning his experiment with these plants at a conference in 1959. Later in life, he allowed a film crew to record his re-creation of Porta's recipe. The fullest account of Peuckert's experiment is given in Johanna Micaela Jacobsen's 2007 Ph.D. dissertation (University of Pennsylvania): "Boundary Breaking and Compliance: Will-Erich Peuckert and 20th Century German Volkskunde."

MODERN-DAY FLYING OINTMENTS FOR MEDICINAL AND RITUAL USE

Today, flying ointments and ritual entheogens are making a comeback in the practice of modern witchcraft. They are a multipurpose tool used for divination, speaking with the dead, traveling to other worlds to retrieve knowledge, and working with the spirit realm. For many years, ritual entheogens were equated with hallucinogenic drugs in the modern neo-pagan community, and knowledge of these plants returned to the shadows. Their lore survived in folk magic and traditional witchcraft circles.

These preparations are being sought out as a means of achieving altered states of consciousness and inducing trance to connect with deities and nature spirits, practice shape-shifting, and acquire information psychically. Achieving hallucinogenic doses is not the goal here, and with most of these plants, the hallucinogenic dose and toxic dose are precariously close. At safe dosages, these preparations can provide a means for enhancing altered states in combination with other techniques. They relax the body and mind, lowering inhibitions and opening the practitioner up to subtle reality.

Making a Flying Ointment

Flying ointments are easy to make in theory, and one can use any basic salve-making recipe. Salves are made by infusing oil with dry plant material and then heating the oil along with beeswax to give it a thicker consistency. Vitamin E oil or rosemary essential oil can be added to help with preservation. I use grapeseed oil because it already contains vitamin E and is practically scentless, but any vegetable oil will work. You can also take a more traditional route and use rendered pork or goose fat.

Other essential oils can also be added for aromatherapy or to enhance the action of the ointment. Mugwort essential oil can be added if you plan on using the ointment for divination or to enhance dreaming and produce more vivid experiences if applying the ointment before bed. Clary sage, lavender, rosemary, and spikenard all have the effect of enhancing the mental faculties, dream recall, and mental clarity. This helps with keeping focused and bringing information back from the spirit world.

Some practitioners will also add additional ingredients for their sympathetic magic. Animal remains can be added to incorporate the power and guidance of the animal's spirit. Goose feathers or crow feathers can be burned and the ashes added to increase the power of transvection or soul flight. Powdered toad skin or the shed skins of snakes can be used to create ointments particularly for shape-shifting and for their connection to occult knowledge and cunning craft. When adding animal remains like this, make sure they are finely powdered and only use minute amounts. This addition is sympathetic, and larger amounts are not necessary.

Soot was a common ingredient listed in medieval flying ointment recipes. Some people theorize that it was to darken the ointment so that the witch could see where it was applied and how much was used. A more scientific explanation suggests that the alkalinity of organic ash helps with the transdermal absorption of the alkaloids. Adding the ashes of certain woods for their magical correspondence allows for a wide variety of effects. Soot can also be obtained by holding a metal spoon over a candle and scraping off the resulting "lamp black," but this process is time consuming. I prefer using the ashes of stems from the plants I am using or hardwood ash. I use one teaspoon per cup of oil, adding it to the infused oil while it is still warm, before straining the herbs. By using the ashes of the same plant, you are effectively creating an energetically whole ointment, like a spagyric tincture.

When infusing the oil, it is important to use heat because the water-soluble alkaloids do not extract as readily into the oil as they do into water or alcohol. A small amount of vodka can be poured over the dry plant material before infusing. This helps break down the cell walls of the plant and makes the extraction process more efficient. I use a double-boiler method to warm the oil by filling a slow cooker with a couple of inches of water, placing a glass jar containing the oil infusion into the water, and letting it sit for four to six hours. I also allow the oil to infuse naturally, leaving it for an additional two to four weeks, taking advantage of both heat and time. The oil is kept in a warm and dark place. After this period, the oil is strained, and any remaining oil is carefully pressed from the plant matter.

In the following recipe, I add 28 g of dried plant material to 250 ml of oil, which is approximately a 1:10 ratio. The oil can be saved separately and used to make individual batches of ointment as needed.

꿱꿱

Flying Ointment

- *Vodka
- *28 g (1 oz.) *Atropa belladonna*
- *250 ml vegetable oil
- *1 tsp. wood or plant ashes
- *4 Tbsp. beeswax or carnauba wax
- *Essential oils

Pour about one shot of vodka over the dry plant material and mix the oil with the plant material. Infuse this mixture in a saucepan over low heat for four to six hours; optionally, leave to infuse at room temperature for two to four weeks.

Strain the oil into a mason jar and add one teaspoon of ash and four tablespoons of beeswax or carnauba wax. Place the jar in a saucepan of water that reaches about halfway up the jar. Heat on medium high, stirring occasionally, until all the wax is melted. More beeswax or oil can be added to adjust the consistency.

Add any essential oils and pour into containers. This batch of oil can be used to make eight one-ounce jars containing two tablespoons of infused oil and one to two teaspoons of beeswax. Each one-ounce tin would contain the equivalent of 3.5 g of plant material.

Preparing to Use the Ointment: Mind-Set and Setting
Avoid caffeine, nicotine, greasy foods, and meat for twenty-four hours prior to using the ointment. Caffeine and nicotine can inhibit the

effects of tropane alkaloids. Greasy foods high in fat also prevent the absorption of tropane alkaloids. Fasting for twenty-four hours beforehand is also beneficial and intensifies the effects. Some practitioners will fast and partake in a plant diet prior to ritual application of the ointment. This diet consists of taking microdoses of the entheogen to form a connection with its spirit. This can also be achieved using flower essences and can be begun seven to ten days before the ritual, accompanied by fasting and abstinence from sex and alcohol.

The single most important aspect of preparation when using these plants for magical purposes is to do so with a ritual mind-set: ritualizing the application of the ointment and creating an environment that is conducive to magical practice. Chanting and drumming is beneficial to begin altering consciousness before the effects of the entheogen kick in.

The ideal setting is outdoors, especially in the woods where spirits roam freely; however, while being outdoors provides an intense experience, it isn't always safe. Darkness enhances the effects of the experience and the manifestation of visons. If possible, having another person act as a watcher is beneficial. When you are engrossed in the effects of tropane alkaloids, you can forget that you are under the influence of an entheogen. If performing a specific ritual, prepare the space and arrange the altar with the appropriate tools prior to applying the ointment so that there are no distractions.

When you are ready to apply the ointment, massage the area with your hands first to get the blood flowing to the area and to open the pores. Apply one teaspoon at a time after doing an initial patch test to ensure there are no skin sensitivities. Apply the ointment to the soles of the feet, palms of the hands, forehead, and back of the neck and one or several pulse points, such as the temples, wrists, and back of the knees. The pulse points are close to major arteries, and the palms and soles of the feet are porous, which enhances absorption. Applying the ointment over a wider surface area increases the absorption of the alkaloids.

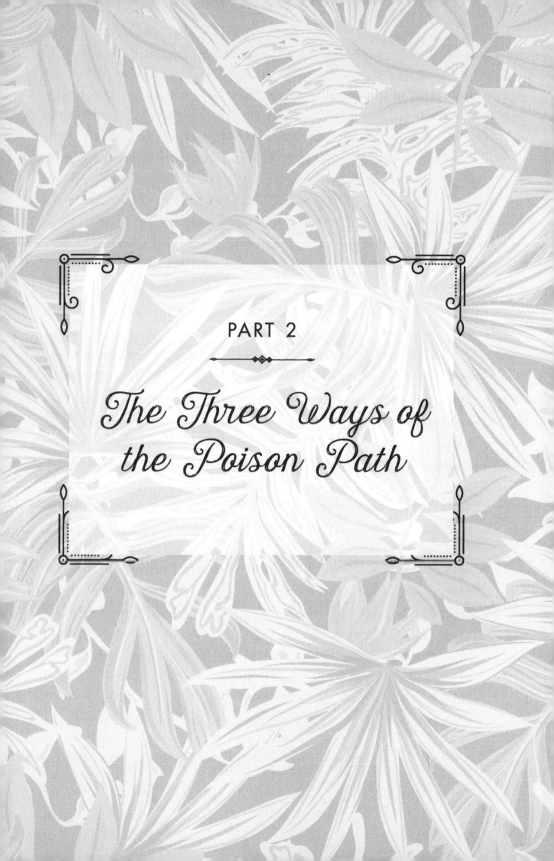

PART 2

The Three Ways of the Poison Path

The Crossroads on the Path of Poison

*T*he division of three forms the foundation for many pagan cosmologies. It reflects the universal divisions of the cycles and laws of nature creation, sustainment, and destruction. The creative forces of the universe being triple in nature are reflected in the Tree of Life and the triangle of manifestation, used by traditional witches; this principle is rooted in the metaphysical belief that the three components of time, space, and energy must come together to manifest something. The triangle is the first geometric shape created by the connection of three points. Triangles can be positioned to gather or direct energy depending on the orientation of their points. Many witches will use a triangle on their altar for this reason.

The kabbalistic Tree of Life also reflects these threefold cycles, with its three spheres at the top arranged in triangular fashion. The supernal forces at the uppermost branches of the tree correspond to the spheres Kether, Binah, and Chokmah. In the triangle, the first and uppermost point is the entirety of the universe, Kether, the divine source. Binah is the void that holds all the potential for creation and life; it is the universal womb. Chokmah is the active perpetuating force; it is the impetus and spark of life that initiates creation. Thus, the image of the Triangle of Arte, also called the Triangle of Solomon, holds the creative forces of the universe.

The triangle, which is the first of the three-dimensional forms, is the

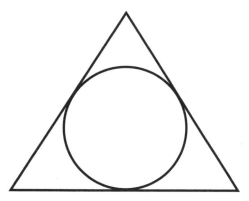

Triangle of Arte, also called the Triangle of Solomon

shape of the planetary force of Saturn, ruling manifestation and crystallization. The top point of the triangle represents the void or source of life. It is the feminine sphere Binah, which is balanced and supported by the male and female representations of divinity as Mercury and Venus. This formation can be used when the nature of the work is celestial, outward, or spiritual in nature. It is the upward-pointing masculine triangle representing the rising flame and active principle.

The inverted triangle positioned on the Tree of Life puts Saturn in the lower realms. In its chthonic aspect, it represents materialization and internalization of spiritual forces, allowing us to go deep within ourselves. Its energy moves in an earthward and inward direction. The properties of balance and structure within this sacred shape are used to create a matrix of spiritual force that is contained therein, concentrating the occult forces raised within the center. The objects or symbols placed within the points of the triangle combine to create a unique synthesis of energies (see the figure on page 38).

CONJURATION AND THE KAMEA

Conjuration is one of the main focuses of the *arte magica*. Utilizing ritual and spell work to access arcane forces to manipulate the movements of nature and redirect the affairs of humankind is the territory of

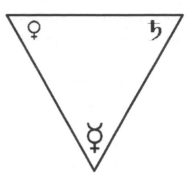

The three ways—
Saturn (top right),
Venus (top left),
Mercury (bottom)

the sorcerer. The craft of the witch makes use of the gifts of nature and strange artifacts that aid her work. Pentacles of Arte, as well as the planetary squares or magic squares known as *kameas* (a Hebrew word meaning "amulet"), can be used to access and imbue objects with planetary forces, drawing them into their corresponding herbs for added potency or when conjuring spirits into objects to enliven them with their power. Placed on the altar within a Triangle of Arte, the kamea is enlivened by chanting, magical gesture, or the sprinkling of powders (see the recipe for an activating powder on page 205). Once activated, the object is placed on the kamea, and similar means are used to concentrate these powers within the object. The figures within the squares represent the numerical resonance of the corresponding planetary body and act as a focal point for its influence (see the figure on page 47).

Working with the Glyphs

A glyph is a pictograph or symbol that expresses in its shape the energy of that which it symbolizes. In this book, glyphs are provided for the baneful herbs (deadly nightshade, black nightshade, bittersweet nightshade, henbane, hemlock, hellebore, mandrake, foxglove, datura, poppy, wolfsbane) as well as for fly agaric. These glyphs can be used for working magic or getting in touch with the spirit of a plant. Drawing the glyph helps focus your mind on the plant you wish to connect with and on your intention.

Light some candles and incense to get into a ritual mind-set. This can be done indoors at your altar or outside. Visualize the plant and express that you want to connect with it. While you are drawing the glyph, recall the qualities of the plant and its history to imbue the glyph with the energy of the plant. Once the glyph is complete, sit in meditation on the glyph and record any flashes of insight you receive during or after this ritual. You can also sleep with the glyph under your pillow to see what comes through in your dreams. That is often how plant spirits communicate with us.

THE THREEFOLD COSMOLOGY IN MYTHOLOGY, WITCHCRAFT, AND ALCHEMY

The threefold cosmology of ancient pagan cultures is found in numerous settings and forms. For example, we see the three cauldrons as energy centers in Celtic mythology; the divisions of land, sky, and sea; and the widespread cosmological divisions of upper, middle, and lower world systems of Norse and Germanic cultures, which have made their way into the modern pagan movement as well as the religion of Wicca. The triangle and triple spiral represent this threefold worldview and have adaptations in Solomonic magic and traditional witchcraft. The archetypal forces of Saturn, Venus, and Mercury are aligned with the currents of magic, witchcraft, and plant lore, providing powerful allies to one's craft.

These three elder forces manifested in the archetypes of the corresponding planets have many things in common, including their chthonic and celestial aspects. Their association with boundaries and liminal spaces in addition to their correlations with the otherworld and witchcraft mythos are the powerful themes expressed in this book.

The three cosmic forces have prominent roles in magical herbalism and the craft of the witch, and when these patterns are recognized, they are undeniable. They represent the traditional core aspects of the witch's practice as a means of discovering, integrating, and using the environment. These archetypes represent the currents of occult forces that practitioners of the craft call upon to advance their knowledge and increase their power. Each force represents a facet of arcane practice and occult knowledge hidden in the natural realm, whether it be the interaction with spiritual powers present in nature or traversing the boundaries between the upper and lower realms for divine inspiration or ancestral wisdom. These are the powers most closely allied with the practice of witchcraft, and understanding their history, mythology, and nuanced connections allows practitioners to connect with the deeper forces beyond their superficial masks.

This book seeks to explore these paths and the entities that we encounter along the way. Through an investigation of these spirits and the plants that are connected to them, we gain a deeper understanding of the powers available to us. The gods and their stories are keys to unlocking the deepest forces of the natural world and those elder spirits recognized by our earliest ancestors. It is where these beings, through their folklore, overlap and the lines between them blur that we can find the greatest insights. It is at the intersection of spirit and myth that we learn the true essence of these changeling gods and goddesses, the deities of witchcraft, science, and medicine.

One thing these three recurring forces of the classical pantheons have in common is their universality and their connection to magic. Their nature is recognizable in numerous ancient pantheons that run deep into the darkest depths of history, going back to Sumerian and Babylonian mythology. These ancient spirits of the Middle East made their way from the fertile black land of Egypt, crossing the Mediterranean and migrating to Europe, where they were reunited with their northern manifestations. The ancient gods of Scandinavia, the British Isles, and those dwelling deep in the forests of central Europe have the same roots. Starting their journey in the cradle of civilization, early nomadic groups spread their worship across the continent where gods and goddesses of similar characteristics and names seemed to have arisen independently, their common origins lost to time and memory.

In the symbolism of alchemy, Saturn, Venus, and Mercury all play prominent roles, each representing one of the three various stages of transmutation. While Saturn represents the first *nigredo* phase of blackening, Venus represents the second *albedo* stage of turning white, and Mercury the final stage of *rubedo* or reddening. The interplay of these three stages comprises the magnum opus or Great Work of the alchemist and the crossroads of the Poison Path.

SATURNUS, THE OLD ONE

Saturnus is a god of great antiquity whose origins are obscure. He is said to be the son of Gaia (or Terra) and Uranus (or Caelus) and the grandchild of Aether and Dies—the most ancient of all gods. Aether, who embodies the pure air of heaven, is by some accounts the son of Erebus (darkness) or Chronos (time), and Dies is the embodiment or goddess of day.

Saturn, one of the Titans, once lived in Olympus and ruled Earth. According to a prophecy, Saturn would be overthrown by one of his sons. To avoid this outcome, he devoured his sons as soon as they were born, but one, Zeus, escaped this fate and later forced Saturn to regurgitate his siblings. Zeus and his siblings deposed Saturn, and Zeus ascended the throne. Exiled from Olympus, Saturn fled to Latium, the land that would become Rome. It is here that he shared the kingdom with Janus—although other accounts say that Saturn had been there all along. He taught the Romans the art of cultivation and agriculture, helping them work the land to release her bounty. The time of Saturn's rule was known as the golden age, when men and beasts lived in harmony and had all that they needed given to them through the bounty of Earth. He was also known for binding the people with "chains of brass" when he taught them the concept of a system of currency. In ancient Rome, it seems he held a much more positive role, acting as benefactor and teacher to humanity, in contrast to the negative reputation he had with the ancient Greeks. Saturnalia, the ancient Roman festival in celebration of Saturn, was originally held on December 17 and later expanded to December 23. During this festival, social norms were inverted, and masters served their slaves in good humor. This feasting and celebration in excess was in remembrance of the bygone golden age of man.

During the Middle Ages, Saturn, the deity and the planet, lost much of his more positive attributes and became known as the greater malefic. He became connected with witchcraft, the devil, and the dark places unknown to mankind. As the last of the visible planets of antiquity, he occupied the border between the known universe and the abyss. He is the great intermediary between the inner solar system and the outer planets.

Astrologically, Saturn rules the sign Capricorn, which begins on the winter solstice. Saturn is present during our most difficult and transformative experiences, which crystallize our will and force us to push ourselves beyond our perceived limitations to where our true purpose lies. On the outer boundary of the inner solar system, his perspective is one of long periods of time and slow movements. He is wise Father Time, who has seen the passing of ages. He is "saturated" with years and sometimes depicted as a wizened old man with a long beard.

VENUS, QUEEN OF THE CRAFT

In magic, sorcery, and green witchcraft, Venus is identified as the feminine counterpart of Mercury. Although the planet most opposite to the forces of Venus is Mars, represented by complete masculinity, aggression, and the iron of Earth, Mercury has more in common with the Witch Star. They are both connected to magical practice and have a transformative planetary movement and multifaceted nature. Like Mercury, Venus has a light and dark aspect, spending part of the year in the morning sky and part of the year in the evening sky. The planet also exhibits phases just like the moon, going through a period of waxing from a sliver to an apogee of fullness and then waning back to a sliver. Many of the goddesses associated with magic are triple in nature, exhibiting these phases, which represent the cycles of life and the ebb and flow of the universe. Venus's triple nature also allows her to exist simultaneously in the three realms. She is the quintessential creatrix, sustainer, and destroyer.

In her position as Morning Star, she is the light bringer who heralds the rising sun. She is Lucifera, the feminine counterpart of Lucifer, bringing the illuminating power of divine wisdom into the waking consciousness. As the Evening Star, she accompanies the sun on its journey into the underworld, casting her starry robes over Earth.

Astrologically, the planet Venus has notable connections to the otherworld and witchcraft in particular. Her path around the sun, when it crosses the orbital path of Earth, creates five points every cycle that, when connected, create a perfect pentagram. She is also connected to the most ancient goddesses of the moon and stars, such as Luna and Ishtar. Like the other manifestations of the Great Goddess, she is both nurturing and destructive, ruling over plants of healing and poison. With her enchantments, she can inspire love and just as quickly take it away. She is a patron of the venereal arts, one of the specialties of the famous Thessalian witches, known for their aphrodisiacs and anaphrodisiacs. Using her knowledge of the plants of the witch's garden, she is credited with the creation of love philters and elixirs of beauty and immortality. The words *veneficus, venefica,* and *venom* all have Venus as their root. To the green practitioner, Venus is an important ally, ruling the fertilization and abundance of the natural world.

MERCURIUS, THE MAGICIAN

Mercurius is the magician, trickster, and shape-shifting shaman. He is credited with gifting humanity with the arts and sciences. Wearing many masks, this progenitor of civilization was also linked to the devil of folklore. He shares much in common with other deities that descended to teach early humans the ways of language and alchemy and the power of symbol. Prometheus, Loki, Lucifer, and Thoth were responsible for delivering the fire of inspiration and craftsmanship to humankind. They are the intermediaries of the spirit world, the material realm, and the abode of the ancestors. Acting as messengers of the gods, they also served as arbitrators, settling many of their disputes.

On the one hand, Mercurius is associated with mediation. He

reasoned with the gods, helping them reach agreements. His words had the attention of Jupiter-Zeus, the king of the gods; he acted as the king's adviser, like Merlin did for King Arthur. Thoth, the Egyptian scribe-god, inventor of writing and magic, played a similar role, arbitrating disputes among the gods and presiding over the judgment of the dead.

On the other hand, Mercurius is associated with tricksters and shape-shifters, using his magic to distort perception, creating chaos among the gods. He is known for his powers of flight and transformation, reflected in the planetary movement of the celestial body bearing the same name. Mercury, the divinity and the planet, is a spirit of dark and light sides. Part of his transit is spent below the horizon, in the underworld and the human subconscious, where the shadow dwells. He then ascends to midheaven and journeys above the horizon, exalting himself as he spends time among the stars and gods of the heavens. This nocturnal and diurnal dance is further transformed by his regular retrograde motion. Like the shaman who dances backward and the witch who walks her circle widdershins to cast spells of blight and call up the shadows, Mercury rains down discord upon Earth four times a year. This change in perspective and forward motion reminds us that there is wisdom in transformation, and repetitive cycles lead to stagnation.

———— ☀ ————

At the crossroads of the Poison Path, the powers of the three realms intersect. The nuanced language of plants and their hidden powers help us uncover the secrets of the most ancient entities that have survived the millennia by changing their masks as their true essence is contained in the lore of the witch. Each of the plants of this path contains a piece of all three of these elder spirits, connected by their roots that are nourished in the depths of the lower realms.

Mercury the magician teaches us how to fly, how to leave our bodies and descend to the depths by changing our shape, flying with wings or slithering into the roots of trees. Venus teaches us to recognize our inner power and our own triple nature. She shows us how to make illusions and enchant the world around us. Where Mercury rules the writing of spells, Venus rules the mixing of potions and ointments that bring us vision and destroy our enemies. Saturn is the great father of it all; he is the witch father and horned master of the wild places. On one side, he is the gatekeeper, the great tree that connects the worlds, and on the other side, he is the devourer of souls who reduces us to our skeletons and reassembles us, thereby marking us.

5

The Book of Saturn
Baneful Herbs and Dark Workings

Saturn acts as the adversary who points out those parts of ourselves that we are afraid to confront, forcing us to embrace our shadow. As the teacher of agriculture and sower of seeds, he is connected with Cain, the first farmer and son of Adam. He wields the scythe, which harvests what is bountiful, discarding the rest. It was Cain who sacrificed his harvest of plants and produce to God, while his brother, Abel, sacrificed the lamb. The opinion that Cain's sacrifice of the crops he had tended by the sweat of his brow was one of dedication and patience, only to be refused by a bloodthirsty god, is one surrounded in controversy. His anger and disappointment at the refusal of his sacrifice was what led him to kill Abel with a blade fashioned from the jaw of a goat. This action forever marked him, and he was condemned to wander Earth as an outsider on the periphery of civilization. Cain is a patron of the work of the traditional witch and the green sorcerer, who specializes in working with plants.

Sigil of the intelligence
of Saturn
(From Agrippa, *Three
Books of Occult Philosophy*)

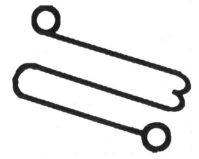

Saturn rules over boundaries, that which separates the civilized world from the wildwood and scorching desert. He rules over wayside plants that grow in the wasteland and those botanical poisons that restrict the life force, pushing the spirit beyond the boundaries of its physical body. In herbalism, Saturn rules over plants with dark leaves, white flowers, and earthy roots. Medicinally, he is associated with the skeleton and muscular system and plants that heal and strengthen the connective tissues and supporting structures of the body. The baneful herbs over which he presides grow in the garden of Hecate, the witch's garden, where noxious herbs of a sinister nature thrive. All of the plants of the Poison Path have an underlying chthonic quality, which puts them in the domain of Saturnus. He is the green devil, the adversarial spirit of nature who has malice for the men who would destroy the ancient forests and sacred groves, forgetting the ancient knowledge of those who lived in harmony with the natural world. This is the spirit of nature that tests those who seek the secrets hidden within Earth. The green devil, the protector and guardian of the natural world, manifests as the old horned god. Like the deep running roots of the ancient forests, his treasures are hidden but well worth the descent into the earth to uncover them. The green devil is a shape-shifter, a changing force exhibiting the powers of both growth and vegetation as well as death and decay. He is a Mercurian spirit with a dark Saturnian side.

The Mercurian plants of shamanic flight allow us to transcend and descend the world tree, while the heavier forces of Saturn and the

4	9	2
3	5	7
8	1	6

Kamea of Saturn
(From Agrippa, *Three Books of Occult Philosophy*)

iron of Mars hold us here by the affinity of our blood with the iron of Earth. This acts as an anchor in our world when we are seeking the chthonic and telluric forces of Earth. In the glyph of Saturn (see the upper right corner of the triangle on page 38), we see the scythe, which cuts through the veil, that invisible membrane between our world and the next, while we remain anchored by the cross of matter. This is the grounding and earthy quality of Saturn, much like the inverted pentagram, which also acts as a gateway.

THE POWER OF SATURN TO COMMUNE AND TRAVEL WITH SPIRITS

Being able to work with the spirits is of paramount importance to classical witchcraft and occult practice. The three classes of spirits are celestial, ancestral, and chthonic and include many overlapping variations of nature spirits. These spirits are all potential teachers along the Crooked Path. This is the path of the green witch, the wort cunner,* and the magical herbalist. It is a middle road, sometimes dark and sometimes light. Just as plants are not inherently malicious or benevolent, one with this knowledge can both heal and harm. The Poison Path reflects this balance, teaching that the line between poison and medicine is often blurred. Deities of witchcraft, ancestors of blood and tradition who also worked these ways, and the spirits that dwell upon and within the land can all be roused through the dark and strange fire of witchcraft.

The powers of Saturn can be used to temper the flame so that it acts as a beacon for specific types of spirits but also as a foundation and container for the ritual. The crystallizing and containing effects of this planetary force, reflected by its many rings, infuse the bounds of our circle with its power, drawing and holding forces within our sacred space. The influence of elemental earth, which corresponds to the heavy

---

Wort cunner is a Middle English term that means plant (wort) knower (from *cunnen,* meaning "to know"). A wort cunner is more than an herbalist; she is someone who knows and works with plant spirits.

nature of Saturn, is also present, allowing for a more material manifestation by providing a denser energy for the spirits to use. The planetary energies can be accessed by the traditional ways of plant, stone, and seal, which provide the physical matrix around which the ritual takes its form. I have used this invocation for calling upon the power of the Old One:

Celestial titan, Saturnian spirit, ringed Kronos, chthonic king of death, heavenly body, thousand-bound giant of the sky, turn your gaze to my terrestrial circle. May your dark might settle here and mingle with the power of my rite.

A power known to all who traffic in the forbidden arts is the ability to leave the body behind in a catatonic-type state, achieved through trance, ritual, and herbal preparation. The ability to travel in spirit to do acts of healing or harm has been used since people first reached out to the spirit world. This power can be used to travel into the realm of spirits and retrieve information or encounter specific forces, such as descent to the underworld for healing or retrieval of ancestral wisdom. Spells cast in spirit form swiftly reverberate throughout the astral realms.

This art also falls under the realm of Saturn as gatekeeper. The baneful herbs that are known as entheogens for their ability to break down barriers between normal consciousness and the spirit world help us easily reach these altered states. Although they act as shortcuts, they also leave us more vulnerable and out of control, putting us at the mercy of those forces we have sought out. Taking these herbs in a micro or therapeutic dose is effective at lowering our conscious barriers, allowing us to more easily achieve trance and spirit flight. The ingestion of these powerful herbs is something too traumatic and dangerous to be done on a regular basis or for recreation and should only be attempted with full understanding under the rarest of circumstances, accompanied by ritual preparation.

THE SEAL AND PENTACLE OF SATURN
FOR WITCHES' WORKINGS

The seal of Saturn and its pentacles from the Book of Solomon are used for their proficiency in those arts classically identified with witchcraft, *maleficium* and *veneficium,* operations specifically under the domain of Saturn. The intelligence of Saturn aids in necromantic works of divination and underworld travel. This is represented by Saturn's planetary glyph, which shows the cross of matter exalted over the crescent of spirit. This can also be seen as a descent, climbing down the roots of the Tree of Life into the lower realms. As a force of restriction and crystallization, the seal can be used to bind someone's actions, call upon someone's karma, or help us work through our own issues with the past. The sickle, a symbol of Saturn, teaches us to cut away the old growth of the previous year. That which no longer serves us can be used as fertilizer for the development of new growth and expansion. Saturn can bring permanency and stability to a magical work that is meant to have long-term effects. Due to its history of being associated with witchcraft and baneful herbs, this planetary energy can be called upon as wise teacher who can bring new insights into practices lost to the past. Saturn can be called upon by witches and the like due to the favorable alignment of the witch's nature and the Saturnian currents.

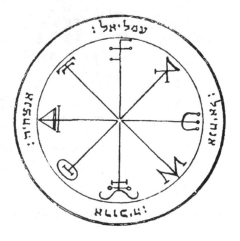

Third pentacle of Saturn from the Key of Solomon. The pentacle should be drawn at the altar in a ritualistic manner. This pentacle is used at night to invoke the spirits of Saturn. The symbols at the ends of the rays in the wheel are the magical characters of Saturn, surrounded by the names of the angels Omeliel, Anachiel, Arauchiah, and Anazachia in Hebrew.

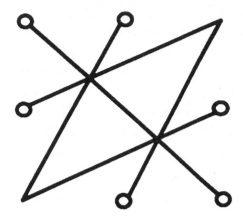

The seal of Saturn
(From Agrippa, *Three Books of Occult Philosophy*)

THE ARCANE ARTS
OF THE POISON PATH

No, no, go not to Lethe, neither twist,
Wolfsbane, tightrooted for its poisonous wine.
Nor Suffer thy pale forehead to be kissed,
By Nightshade, ruby grape of Proserpine.

JOHN KEATS, "ODE TO MELANCHOLY"

The cunning craft of the green sorcerer goes beyond the practices of the botanist and herbalist. Although potent in chemistry, the medicine of the plants associated most closely with magic is a medicine of spirit. The green sorcerer is both a magician and an alchemist who uses her green thumb to unlock the secrets of nature. By cultivating a magical garden, brewing potions, and working with plant spirits, she hones her craft providing powerful medicine for others. The plants of the green sorcerer are influenced both by the celestial rays of the planets as they dance across the sky and by elemental currents that manifest in their physical characteristics and chemical components. It is the dark-green fire of Earth, the hidden telluric currents that we seek to connect with on the path. It is our focus on the chthonic and creative forces of the land and its spirits that is quintessential to this practice.

The Poison Path unites the art of green sorcery, alchemy, and spirit work into a unique synthesis incorporating various currents of magic and myth. One of the main goals of the green witch is to facilitate the same familiar relationships with spirits of the plant realm as one would with any other familiar or tutelary spirit. As with any such relationship, one must first introduce oneself and become accustomed to the particularities of the individual spirit, such as their characteristics, methods of operation, and various affinities for specific offerings and modes of working.

Plant spirits, in particular, are naturally aligned with the practice of magic. Often blurring the lines between bewitchment and medicine, as teachers these ancient entities have much to show us beyond the realms of stem and seed. The plants themselves are in direct connection with the Earth and its subterranean networks of energy and consciousness. Those plants that are associated with spirit communication, night flights, and devilish forces in general gained their reputations through their strange otherworldly presence and powerful actions on the human body and mind.

Plants communicate in a way that is beyond words and images and that is still not understood by human science. However, over time and through repeated contact, the subtle language of plants can begin to be understood by those who work with their spirits on a regular basis. The bodies of plants are physical manifestations of the unseen forces of nature and the interplay of occult energies within the Earth. As such, they are able to communicate complex ideas and desires to the gods and spirits via their symbolism and inherent properties. The symbolic folklore accumulated by a specific group of plants over time is a container for the plants' specific type of energy. Through the understanding of correspondence and the doctrine of signatures, we are able to tap into and combine these energies with our own in unique ways to achieve powerful effects.

By working with these plants in their living state, whether in the wild or in the witch's garden, one begins to gain an intimate understanding of the plant's nature through observing its behavior and life cycle.

HERBS OF SATURN

Belladonna · Black Nightshade · Eastern Black Nightshade · Bittersweet Nightshade · Black Henbane · Poison Hemlock · Black Hellebore · Mugwort · Wormwood · Agrimony · Solomon's Seal

Physical Characteristics

The following characteristics are drawn from *The Complete Herbal* by Nicholas Culpeper, a seventeenth-century herbalist, astrologer, and physician.

Leaves: hairy, hard, dry, parched, coarse, and of ill-favored appearance

Flowers: unprepossessing, gloomy, dull, greenish, faded or dirty white or pale red, prickly, and disagreeable

Roots: spreading widely in the earth, rambling around in discursive fashion

Odor: fetid, putrid, and muddy

Medicinal Properties

The plants of Saturn affect the connective tissues, the skeleton, and the teeth. They also help the body process minerals, assisting in their absorption. Saturnian herbs can be used for shielding, protection, endurance, restriction, and self-control. Spiritually and emotionally, they can help us make necessary changes in our lives, teaching us to let go and move forward. Working with Saturnian plants give us the fortitude to transcend limitations and begin living our true purpose. Since Saturn is about structure and foundation, plants ruled by this planet help us develop structure and ground ourselves so that we can manifest our desires in the real world. They are typically masculine in nature, grounding, astringent, and cold, with little moisture. They limit chaotic and overflowing energy when one area of our lives is overstimulated. Saturn is a planet of boundaries, and its herbs prevent the spread of bacteria and help heal wounds, mend tissue, and strengthen the bones. Saturnian herbs are particularly beneficial for arthritis pain and back issues.

Astrological Correspondences

The following correspondences are drawn from *Practical Astrology for Witches and Pagans* by Ivo Dominguez Jr. (Dominguez 2016, 64).

> **Capricorn:** cardinal earth
>
> **Tenth House:** prestige, honor, career, the legacy a person leaves behind, attainments necessary to reach life purpose
>
> **Aquarius:** fixed air
>
> **Eleventh House:** belief structures, ideologies, group traditions, how our spirituality is grounded in the community and the world around us

Alchemical Symbolism: Nigredo

This is the first phase of the Great Work, represented by the raven, the black crow, and the toad. It is a process of darkness, of the black sun or the eclipse, when matter is broken down. Spiritually, it can be thought of as the destroying of the ego or the dark night of the soul. It is a spiritual death. This stage is ruled over by Saturn and is known as putrefaction. This is when we begin our journey with the shadow, contacting it for the first time.

Belladonna (*Atropa belladonna*): The Beautiful Seductress

One of the first plants that initially attracted me to the study of herbs connected to witches and magic was *Atropa belladonna,* also called deadly nightshade and the devil's berry. In my own practice, belladonna is a plant spirit ally, a teacher, and a familiar. The air of mystery and intrigue that surrounds this plant is seductive. Her dark-green foliage and deep purple flowers give her a shadowy appeal. Her shiny black berries whisper temptingly that they have many secrets for those willing to risk her deadly kiss. Her influence has spread across cultures; she has fought and won many battles and has many names. Belladonna, as she is commonly called today, was known as banewort, devil's herb, great morel, and tolkirsche. Belladonna was also known as dwale berry. The English word *dwale* comes from a Scandinavian root word meaning "trance" and was also a synonym for a sleeping potion made using *Atropa belladonna*. In the medical community, her name underwent changes as well; she was known as *Solanum lethale* until 1788 and was reintroduced as *Belladonna folia* in 1809.

Her relatives, the mandrake, henbane, and thorn apple, comprise the family of great witching herbs. These plants have shown up throughout antiquity as powerful medicines and in the apothecaries of the oldest witches of legend. The plants of the Solanaceae family were known for their sedative and pain-relieving properties and also for their powers of vision and spirit flight. There are other less common varieties of the nightshade family, such as the more potent yellow belladonna (*Atropa belladonna* var. *lutea*) and the devilish-looking Russian belladonna, also known as henbane bell (*Scopolia carniolica*). These beautiful varietals have a most otherworldly look and are coveted by enthusiasts of baneful herbs.

Belladonna in History and Mythology

Belladonna is sacred to the goddess Hecate, who was so feared and respected as a Titan goddess that when the gods took over Mount Olympus, Zeus gave her rule over the sea, sky, and underworld. Belladonna's martial qualities are evident in her connection to her namesake Bellona, the Roman goddess of war, and are reflected in the plant's unpredictability. She can be fashioned into a powerful fetish of protection in spiritual warfare and used to empower weapons for physical protection and spiritual battle. In this aspect, Belladonna is a warrior goddess, sovereign of the battlefield. She is like the Morrígan (meaning "great queen" or "phantom queen"), the Irish goddess of war and fate who flies above the battlefield, much like the Valkyrie, Norse maidens who collect the souls of fallen warriors. Belladonna was known as Walkerbeeren (Valkyrie berry) or Walkerbaum (Valkyrie tree) in northern Europe.

Her Venusian aspects are also well placed on the battlefield. History has shown us the power that feminine nature commands to turn the tides of war. With their words and charms, women raise and inspire armies and have themselves led them into victory. The fierce female spirits of the battlefield collect the souls of those who died honorably. Women often win wars with cunning and discipline. This type of cunning has brought victory to those who would have otherwise been outmatched by brute force. Belladonna was used in the eleventh century by the Scots under King Duncan I, who gave the invading Danish army belladonna-infused beer. Once weakened by delirium, they were easily overpowered. The plant is also thought to have been used in the Parthian Wars to poison the troops of Marcus Antonius. Plutarch gives a detailed account of the poison's strange effects (Grieve 1971).

Manipulation, coercion, and espionage are also a means of ensuring victory and are among the powers of this plant. Belladonna has a seductive and hypnotic quality that can be used in charms of commanding and compelling. Her abilities can bend an iron will and bring it under one's control. Her darker aspects show us how to use subversive means to achieve our ends, by working in the shadows. Her Venusian qualities temper her martial aspects, which can destroy all in their path. She is a spirit of secrets and illusions, keeping things hidden from her enemies while exposing truths that would cripple their success.

Her Latin name refers to Atropos, one of the three Fates believed responsible for cutting the thread connecting one to the web of life. Like Atropos, the fate who cuts the cord of life, Saturn also rules separation, an action that appears in this plant's ability to separate us from our bodily fluids and in some cases our life force. While Mercury is the traveler who goes between realms, Saturn is the gatekeeper found at all boundaries, holding all keys to the otherworld. In this capacity gatekeeper herbs like belladonna can be called upon to cut a window or door through the veil. While Mercurian plants allow us to transform and grow wings to travel above and below, Saturnian plants open the way here in the middle realm. Just as the pupils are opened to resemble the dark void of the belladonna berry, our inner world is opened as well.

Belladonna, the beautiful lady, was an infamous herb used in the Middle Ages by physicians and magicians alike. It is mentioned in many obscure and well-known manuscripts on medicine and medieval books on magic. The plant was used in common medicinal preparations into the 1800s before eventually fading into obscurity, its medicinal and magical value remembered only by herbalists and cunning folk. Today, she is reclaiming her infamy in the lore of classical witchcraft and modern entheogenic study. Her name was once known across Europe, and she went by many sinister titles.

Hildegard von Bingen (1098–1179 CE), in an effort to demonize the former heathen ritual plants, wrote of the plant's sinister nature in *Physica:* "The Deadly Nightshade has coldness in it, and this coldness also holds evil and barrenness, and in the earth and at the place where it grows, a diabolic influence has some share and participation in its craft. And it is dangerous for a man to eat or drink, for it destroys his spirit as if he were dead" (Hildegard 1998, 75). Giambattista della Porta lists belladonna as an herb used to shape-shift into an animal, referring to the plant as *Solanum somniferum* (sleeping nightshade).

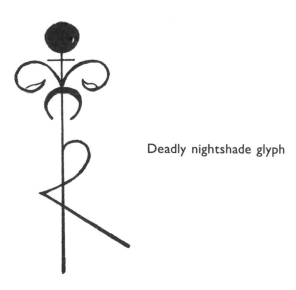

Deadly nightshade glyph

Belladonna in Magical Practice

If one plant spirit were marked as a witch, it would be the spirit of *Atropa belladonna*. Like Hecate, the queen of the witches, belladonna holds a similar status as one of the ruling herbs of the Poison Path. She is a quintessential representation of what it is to be a witch—marked as an outsider, feared for her dangerous nature, and sought out for her powers of glamour and seduction. She is one of the patron herbs of witchcraft and sorcery, and the gifts this plant has to share are manifold, given only to those who approach her with the reverence and respect that she commands. The devil's herb, as she is sometimes called, is an ally to those on the Crooked Path, but make no mistake, she is a harsh teacher to those bold enough to explore her mysteries. The powers that her spirit has collected over the centuries—powers gained from both pagan practice and medieval folklore—take many forms. The diabolism perpetuated in the Middle Ages has only served to expand her already vast repertoire of legendary powers.

As a gatekeeper plant, belladonna opens the energy centers and expands awareness to spiritual realms. She opens gateways to other realms of consciousness, trance, and the otherworld. She can also help us by removing toxic situations and people (Saturn) and providing offensive protection (Mars). Belladonna is a combination of Saturnian energy, being a poisonous plant, and Martian force, due to her aggressive and protective nature. At times she acts as an herb of Venus, with her seductive qualities.

Belladonna is appropriate for works of necromancy, specifically calling the dead to the middle world for assistance. Personal experience recommends employing appropriate protective measures before attempting this. Her affinity with witchcraft makes her a perfect plant for offerings and summoning the mighty dead. She can connect with and reach out to those individuals who have walked the Crooked Path before us and have chosen to remain behind to help other practitioners, thereby continuing their own work.

As a charm, fetish, or talisman, belladonna has numerous applications within the realm of natural magic. The ways this plant can be used to create vessels for spirits or talismans of protection barely scratches the surface of the practical magical applications for this power-enhancing herb. The spirit of the plant also guides the practitioner to new and insightful uses for the plant material.

The aid of this plant as a magical catalyst is matched by few, perhaps rivaled only by her sister nightshades the mandrake, thorn apple, and henbane. As a witch's power plant, she can be added to any formula or charm for added power, specifically when connected to the power of the witch's familiar spirit. As an herb of mastery, this plant can be used to bring success to all one's endeavors. She is known for destroying her enemies by subversive means, binding their actions and exposing their secrets.

Her martial associations with goddesses of war and berserker rage ensure success in offensive magic. She is particularly appropriate for magical warfare, lending her martial qualities and berserker rage to magical weapons when enchanting them. The juice from the berries or leaves can be used to anoint objects of magical protection, divination, and necromantic fetishes. It can also be made into a tincture for the same purposes, which lasts indefinitely.

Medicinal Uses of Belladonna

Belladonna and other solanaceous plants were used to treat many conditions before modern advances in medicine. These plants have also been used for centuries in Eastern herbalism before making their way into medieval Europe. For example, Indian ayurvedic medicine, which has been in practice for thousands of years, uses many of these plants. Ayurvedic tradition suggests that a daily dose of *Atropa belladonna* can be taken medicinally when properly prepared. The suggested daily dosage is 50 to 100 mg of the powdered leaves or 25 to 100 mg of the powdered root per day. Juice from the leaves may be administered in doses of one to four drops taken two or three times a day under the instruction of a professional herbalist.

The leaves have been smoked and were once used in cigarettes to help with asthma. One treatment used up until the early 1900s was called Asthmador, a preparation made by the R. Schiffman Company, comprised of belladonna, datura, and potassium perchlorate. It was sold as cigarettes and in the form of a powder that was burned as incense. When ingested, the powder would cause hallucinations. Infusions of the plant when ingested are sure to cause the uncomfortable drying up of the body's fluids, resulting in an extremely dry mouth and an inability to urinate, which lasts long after the plant has been ingested.

Historically, the plant material was used in plasters, poultices, and ointments for pain, and this is a safer way of working with this plant. With their seductive and hypnotic quality, the berries have been used in tinctures and alcohol infusions to induce trance and act as aphrodisiacs that inhibit the senses. The classical lore of Italian women using the tincture to dilate their pupils, which was said to make them look more receptive to amorous affairs, is well known.

Some sources say that the berries may be added to wine, which can be taken in small amounts for its trance-inducing effects for those desiring prophetic visions and contact with the spirit world. It is said that one or two berries will cause minor perceptual changes when ingested, while three or four berries act as a psychoactive with aphrodisiac effects. A hallucinogenic dose would be four to nine berries, while anything higher would be fatal in an adult. There are accounts of children being accidentally poisoned after eating just two or three berries. Dioscorides, a Greek physician and pharmacologist whose work *De Materia Medica* was the leading pharmacological text for over a thousand years, wrote extensively on these plants. He recorded that one drachm (3.4 g) of the root infused in wine was enough to bring about hallucinations. Four grams or more would cause death.

This gives us an idea of the unpredictable nature of this plant. On the one hand, it can be used as an effective analgesic and anesthetic, while on the other hand, it can easily take one's life. The belladonna alkaloids were responsible for the death of Robert Cochrane, a practitioner who devoted much study to this plant.* There are many factors that can cause the alkaloids in this plant to increase, and certain methods of preparation will extract them more effectively than others.

Great care should be taken with any entheogenic preparation; it should be prepared with reverence for the powerful plants being invoked. This is especially true for plants of a sinister Saturnian nature. Ingestion of belladonna causes dilation of the pupils and blurred vision, sleep plagued by strange dreams, and delusions in the waking state in which one is unaware that one is under its effects due to the amnesiac effects of scopolamine. The effects of this plant vary widely depending on dosage, individual biochemistry, and the method of ingestion. Dilution and gradual increase of dosage, starting with a very small amount, is the safest way to determine the effects the plant will have on one's unique body chemistry.

When used too frequently, tropane alkaloids can build up in the tissues of the heart, resulting in health problems. The unpredictability of belladonna's alkaloids makes it dangerous to ingest orally. There are much safer ways of employing this plant in ritual, and that is the focus of this work. Ingesting any plant containing poisonous alkaloids is not recommended, and the dosages given in the following section are strictly for research purposes.

Belladonna Dosages and Preparation

Chemically, belladonna has a high alkaloid content; her main compounds are atropine (dl-hyoscyamine), solanine, and scopolamine. These tropane alkaloids are the active components for which the plant is known, acting on the human nervous system.

---

*Cochrane was a pivotal figure in the modern witchcraft movement and the magister of the clan of Tubal Cain, a coven of traditional witches. Cochrane allegedly committed ritual suicide on midsummer 1966 with a combination of *Atropa belladonna* and benzodiazepines. Through his last correspondences, we can piece together Cochrane's final few weeks. For more information on the life and death of Robert Cochrane, see *A Poisoned Chalice: The Death of Robert Cochrane* by Gavin Semple.

Belladonna has been used in unconventional ways for its mind-altering properties. There is a tradition in southern Germany where hunters would ingest three or four berries to sharpen their senses. The effectiveness of this practice is reinforced in Morocco, where the dried berries are made into a tea taken with sugar to ease depression and in small doses to clear the mind for intellectual performance. It is also used as a male aphrodisiac (Venzlaff 1977, cited in Rätsch 2005, 83). The leaves and berries have been used in smoking blends combined with *A. muscaria,* and in incense blends for trance and divination.

Belladonna is used in homeopathic medicine to treat anxiety, feelings of distress and uneasiness, heat-related facial flushing, throbbing in the head, nervousness and excitability, and restless sleep plagued by nightmares and for cold extremities and a warm head. The homeopathic dose is a diluted extract not exceeding one part per hundred, according to homeopathic pharmacopoeias, with a total alkaloid content below 0.001 percent. It is used on the basis that the alkaloid content in the mother tincture* is limited to the amount of 0.1 percent alkaloids; 1:100 dilution contains a maximum 0.001 percent (0.01 mg/ml).

In human plasma the half-life of the alkaloids is thirteen to thirty-eight hours. Alkaloids from belladonna preparations are quickly absorbed through the gastrointestinal tract, and transdermal absorption is moderate. Herbivores are much more resistant to the alkaloids than carnivores.

Effects on the human central nervous system may occur in doses of 3 mg atropine or more; 100 mg of atropine in human adults is considered the minimum lethal dose; 10 mg or more of hyoscyamine can be lethal (EMA 1998). The overall main alkaloid is hyoscyamine, at 87.6 percent in leaves, and it racemizes into atropine when extracted or dried. In vitro (in solution), hyoscyamine undergoes rapid racemiza-

---

*The mother tincture is the first stage in creating a homeopathic remedy, before being diluted. It is the base for creating a homeopathic remedy.

tion into atropine. The entire plant contains between 0.272 and 0.511 percent tropane alkaloids. The stalk can contain up to 0.9 percent alkaloids, the unripe berries are 0.8 percent, the ripe berries can range from 0.1 to 9.6 percent, and the seeds are about 4 percent (Lindequist 1992, cited in Rätsch 2005, 83–84).

Medicinal Dosages

Therapeutic dose: 0.05–0.1 g of dried and powdered leaves

Maximum single dose: 0.2 g of herb (corresponds to 0.6 mg of total alkaloids)

Maximum daily dose: 0.6–1.8 mg of total alkaloids

Median single dose: 0.5–1 g of herb (corresponds to 0.15–0.3 mg of total alkaloids)

Mild psychoactive dose: 30–200 mg of leaves or 30–120 mg of dried root

British Pharmacopoeia Dosages

1–2 grains powdered leaves

1–5 grains powdered root

1–3 drops fluid extract of the herbage/aerial parts

¼–1 drop fluid extract of the roots

5–15 drops tincture

5–15 drops juice

Deadly Nightshade Tincture
(Church and Church 2009)

- 1 part *Atropa belladonna* leaves
- 10 parts 70 percent alcohol

Only the leaves are used, harvested in early summer. Cut the leaves from the stem and chop coarsely. Macerate the plant material in alcohol for ten to fourteen days. Dose is 2.5–10 ml per week.

COMMON NIGHTSHADES

Three other varieties of nightshade can be found easily throughout North America, growing in wooded areas, borderlands, and overgrown plots of land. They are black nightshade (also called garden nightshade or European black nightshade), eastern black nightshade (also called West Indian nightshade), and bittersweet nightshade (also called woody nightshade or creeping nightshade). Like all the members of the nightshade family, they have strong connections to magic, the dead, and the spirit world. The first two—*Solanum nigrum* and *Solanum ptychanthum*—are closely related.

❀

Black Nightshade (*Solanum nigrum*), Eastern Black Nightshade (*Solanum ptychanthum*): The Toad Plants

Black nightshade (*Solanum nigrum*)—also known, more obscurely, as petty morel and yerba mora—grows abundantly in unkempt overgrown areas and woodlands. It closely resembles the potato plant with its white flowers and similar leaves and can be used to tap into the same currents as the harder-to-procure and more dangerous sisters of the nightshade family. It is often confused with belladonna or deadly nightshade, the main difference being that deadly nightshade berries grow singly whereas in black nightshade they grow in clusters. *Solanum nigrum* is native to Eurasia but has been naturalized in other parts of the world. The white flowers are slightly larger than in other varieties, and the leaves are wavy or toothed. The plant has been listed in flying ointment recipes, and there is some allusion to it having psychoactive properties.

Solanum ptychanthum (West Indian nightshade or eastern black nightshade) is native to all parts of North America except for the westernmost states. It is a close relative of *Solanum nigrum*. The flowers resemble small white stars. The unripe green berries are toxic; they turn black when they are ripe and are then safe to eat in small amounts.

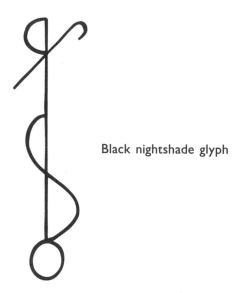

Black nightshade glyph

Solanum spp. can be used in all forms of Hecatean and Saturnian rites associated with the underworld, baneful magic, the dark moon, crone goddesses, and Samhain rituals. The berries are reminiscent of belladonna berries and can also be made into an ink that is useful in spells of binding and protection as well as drawing Saturn's planetary glyphs and pentacles.

Boiling the leaves will remove most of the alkaloids. An infusion of the stems and leaves can be used in weather magic, specifically to bathe rain-making effigies. The leaves can also be dipped in water and used as an aspergillum for rituals of banishing and sympathetic rituals for calling the rain.

Author and herbalist Harold Roth has described these Saturnian, watery plants in a unique way, calling them "toad plants." They were once grown in cottage gardens to provide shade for toads. Henbane, fern, and dandelion are also associated with toads, storms, and the fertile underworld.

Plants belonging to the nightshade family have an affinity for the stone onyx, which resembles the shiny black berries of black nightshade and deadly nightshade. The plant and stone can be stored together to enhance each other's energies, since they are in correspondence with one another.

৵৶

Ensorceled Ink Using Black Nightshade and Deadly Nightshade

The black berries of Solanum nigrum *lose some of their alkalinity as they become ripe, unlike the berries of* Atropa belladonna, *which remain poisonous. Both berries can be used to create ink or dye that imparts its dark qualities into the symbols and words it is used to inscribe. Most of the berries used for the ink in this recipe are black nightshade, with two or three belladonna berries added for their magical potency. The ashes of these plants may be added as well. Grain alcohol is used to make a tincture of the berries. Vinegar can also be used to extract the dyes from the fruits of these plants. Gum arabic (also called acacia gum) is added to achieve the desired consistency, and benzoin tincture may be added for preservation.*

- 2 oz. grain alcohol or vodka
- 1 Tbsp. black nightshade berries
- 2–3 belladonna berries
- Gum arabic
- 15 drops benzoin tincture

To make the ink, you are essentially making an alcohol extract or tincture. Combine the alcohol and plant material and allow the mixture to macerate until a dark color is achieved. Strain out the plant material and add gum arabic. Heat the mixture using a slow cooker or double boiler until the resin is dissolved and the desired consistency is achieved. Add the benzoin tincture before bottling.

India ink may also be added to create a deeper-black ink that may be used for scrying. The ink can be poured on the surface of liquid in a scrying vessel to create a dark liquid mirror. It can also be poured in small amounts and the shapes of the ink may be interpreted. This makes a good medium for scrying with the aid of ancestral spirits or other beings of a shadowy or chthonic nature.

The ink as a writing tool may be used like any other ink for writing sacred alphabets, drawing sigils, and recording spells. This ink is specifically potent for workings of the dark moon and can be used in binding, banishing, or blasting spells, using a thorn as the writing utensil for added potency.

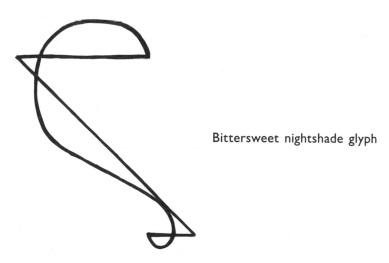

Bittersweet Nightshade (*Solanum dulcamara*): Setting Boundaries

This vining nightshade, also called woody nightshade, grows on a woody stem that each season grows longer and longer. It shares the same dark associations with its family members. This plant is both Saturnian and Mercurian, with influences of earth and air. It corresponds to the underworld aspect of Mercury, Mercurius Psychopompos.

Its entangling and twining growing habits make it a great plant for binding and setting boundaries. The fresh stems can be wrapped around poppets or made into circlets and allowed to dry before being used in ritual. It can be hung in bundles over entryways and in areas where protection is needed. The stems, which become woodier with age, can be cut and bundled with rosewood and iron nails as a protective talisman. The root of the woody nightshade grows large and spreads through rhizomes. It can be harvested and kept as a plant spirit fetish. When placed

Bittersweet nightshade glyph

on the altar it helps obscure the workings from those who would under-mine our operations. It helps with connection to the shadow realm and with integration of the shadow self.

Bittersweet nightshade has been used to protect children and live-stock. Its berries were strung on thread to make a necklace, worn to protect against malicious gossip. The berries can be used in transforma-tive magic, especially lycanthropic magic. To curse an enemy, write the person's name on a dry nightshade stem and lay it at his or her door (Magister Botanicus 1995, cited in Rätsch 2005, 477).

The flowers are a purple color with a bright yellow stamen, and when they turn to berries, they transition from green to yellow and then red. The ripe red berries make good offerings for the spirits of the dead and the Great Goddess in her underworld aspects. They symbol-ize blood, rebirth, and immortality. Resembling drops of blood, they represent ancestral power and the regenerative feminine force of Earth. This nonhallucinogenic relative of the deadly nightshade can be used to explore the crooked ways of the Poison Path, reflected by the spindly growth pattern of this vine. Goddesses such as Hecate, Lilith, Kali, and Inanna all respond to the chthonic nature of this plant, which grows up from the shadows of the forest floor, making its home in the hedge and under the dark boughs of pine trees.

An alchemical motto by fifteenth-century alchemist Basilius Valentinus is contained in its acronym VITRIOL: *Visita Interiora Terrae Rectificando Invenies Occultum Lapidem.* Translated into English it reads: Visit the innermost zones of the earth and by rectification shall you discover the hidden stone. By following the winding vine of *Solanum dulcamara* from the depths of the earth, you are led to the blood-red berries, reminiscent of the blood-red color of the philoso-pher's stone. Descending to the underworld to retrieve arcane wisdom is an important practice of the Poison Path.

Bittersweet nightshade contains approximately 0.3 to 3.0 percent steroidal alkaloids in the herbage and 1.4 percent in the roots. The alkaloid content of the berries declines as they ripen; they eventu-ally become almost completely devoid of alkaloids (Teuscher 1994, cited in Rätsch 2005, 477). One of its main alkaloids is solanine, a steroidal glycoside. It is considered to be the "sleeping strychnos" of Dioscorides, and there are mentions of its use as a sedative narcotic.

༺༻

Home Protection Wreath

This wreath can be made in the summer and allowed to dry and hang all year long. It uses the protective, binding, and banishing properties of bittersweet nightshade to create a protective boundary around your home. As a bonus, it is also said to protect against lightning strikes.

- 3 pieces of three-foot-long bittersweet nightshade vines
- Black thread
- Protective charms or herbs (optional)

Twist together the three vines to form a ring, using black thread to secure it where needed. You can include protective charms and even add other protective herbs to create a larger wreath if desired. Hang the wreath so that it dries completely, but don't hang it outside where it will get wet.

🌱

Black Henbane (*Hyoscyamus niger*): Herb of Twilight Sleep

Henbane is one of the grand herbs of witchcraft, and she is also one of the three fates of the Poison Path, along with her sisters belladonna and mandrake. This is a plant that has a long history of use in shamanism, magic ritual, and associations with the devil, which were acquired during the Middle Ages. The use of henbane in arcane workings goes back hundreds of years prior to the medieval superstitions attached to such plants. Ancient Egyptian knowledge of henbane is documented in the Ebers Papyrus, circa 1500 BCE (Schultes, Hofmann, and Rätsch 1992, 86). This is likely Egyptian henbane (*Hyoscyamus muticus*), known for its higher alkaloid content.

Hyoscyamus niger is a member of the nightshade family, and like its relatives, it contains characteristics of the three planets most associated with magic, sorcery, and the spirit world: Venus, Mercury, and Saturn—the three ways at the crossroads of the Poison Path and three prongs on the witches' trident. This three-pronged categorization can be crudely divided as the dark workings of Saturn, the arts of Venus, and the shamanic arts of Mercury. Within these three groupings, we find the classical arts associated with the practice of witchcraft before the modern witchcraft movement.

This is an herb of the chthonic side of Mercury, the dark aspect of the psychopomp who leads the dead into the underworld. As Mercury can alternate between the light and dark, the upper world and lower world, we are able to follow Mercury to these realms to communicate and retrieve information. This is mirrored in the movement of the planet, which spends part of its orbit in the morning sky and part of it in the night sky. Henbane, like Mercury, can bridge the gap between the living and the dead, and as an offering in necromantic rites, it facilitates this type of divination.

Henbane has traditionally been used as incense, a smoking herb, or a ritual fumigant. It can also be added to beer or wine to increase its intoxicating effects. Shaman's snuff is another way that the powers of this plant can be employed. When the leaves are finely powdered, a small amount can be insufflated via the nostrils for its trance-inducing effects. The seeds have the most consistent alkaloid content and are generally sprinkled on charcoal as offerings to the dead and to release their intoxicating fumes. One way of using the seeds in this manner is to place burning charcoal in a fireproof bowl, sprinkle approximately twenty crushed seeds on it, and cover the bowl with a cloth, allowing the smoke to collect. During the ritual at the appropriate time, the cloth cover is pulled away, allowing a thick cloud of smoke to be inhaled by the practitioner. Albertus Magnus claimed that henbane was used by sorcerers to see daemons and other spirits in its smoke and thus can be used as a medium for manifestation and scrying.

Henbane is one of the hexing herbs, a group of plants with an affinity with witches and their craft. In a Pomeranian witchcraft trial in 1538, an accused witch confessed to giving a man henbane seeds to make him "crazy" with sexual arousal. In another trial of the Inquisition, one of the accused divulged her technique for separating two lovers, which she did by strewing henbane seeds between them, while incanting, "Here I sow wild seed, and the Devil advised that they would hate and avoid each other until these seeds had been separated" (Marzell 1922, cited in Rätsch 2005, 278).

As one of the earliest herbs of necromantic and funerary rites, henbane seeds have been found in Neolithic funerary vessels buried with the dead. Hercules was said to wear a crown of henbane and poplar leaves, which signified his ability to travel to the underworld and back. The newly returning dead were also crowned with a circlet of henbane when crossing the River Lethe, the henbane intended to cause them to forget the toils of their former lives.

In Greek mythology, henbane was named *herba Apollinaris*, after the god Apollo and his oracle at Delphi. It was burned and smoked for its visionary effects, opening the gates of the upper and lower worlds. It is also a powerful herb of consecration, particularly for spirit vessels, tools of divination, and relics of shamanic travel intended to be taken to the spirit world.

Henbane's Latin name comes from the Greek *hyoskyamos*, which means "hog's bean." Pigs are immune to the toxic effects of henbane and are thought to enjoy its inebriating effects. Hyoskyamos is sacred to the underworld goddess Persephone. Some historians think the mythical *nepenthes pharmakon*, a magical potion given to Telemachus and his men by Helen in Homer's *Odyssey* to help them forget their grief, may have contained henbane, a claim refuted by Louis Lewin.

Henbane is sacred to the deities Saturn, Hecate, and Hel and the thunder gods Thor and Donar. Those who rule and dwell in the shadowy realms of the underworld can be summoned using this plant whose smoke acts as a bridge between the realms.

It is said that Germanic witches who were known for their weather magic used the herb in rituals of rain making. The smoke of the plant was thought to cause rain clouds to gather. When used in an infusion to empower weather-working tools, henbane adds its power. The entire plant can be dipped in a body of water and splashed upon a stone, a traditional rain-making practice.

Some sources say that three grams is the maximum daily dose for the medicinal effects of *Hyoscyamus niger*. The herb is still used in ayurvedic medicine, and while the herb contains toxic tropane alkaloids, it has been used for millennia as a soporific (sleep aid) and pain reliever. The seeds are most effective for their use in trance-inducing ritual fumigations due to their consistency in alkaloid content. The leaves, stems and roots may be used in traditional ointments and oils for pain relief, known as oleum henbane. Topical application is much safer than ingesting this plant internally, as with any plant containing tropane alkaloids. Although safer than ingestion, topical application is not without risks and should be approached with caution, starting with an application of a conservative amount in a small area to determine if any adverse reactions occur.

Lewin, in *Phantastica,* describes being under the influence of henbane as a feeling of "pressure in the head, the limbs of the body become heavy and sight is affected becoming vague while images stretch lengthwise." He gives accounts of visual distortions, such as seeing black circles on silver backgrounds or green circles on gold backgrounds (Lewin 1998, 193). According to a description in *Plants of the Gods,* those experiencing henbane intoxication feel a pressure in the head and the eyelids become heavy. Sight is unclear, and objects look distorted; henbane's effects often include disturbing hallucinations (Schultes, Hofmann, and Rätsch 1992, 87).

Henbane in Magical Practice

As a powerful visionary plant, black henbane is widely known for its shamanic and divinatory uses. It has been used by Germanic and Nordic cultures for its intoxicating properties and its power as an aphrodisiac. Henbane and its magical uses are not limited to these cultures, and its use is widespread across Europe and Asia. Its connections to Norse magic

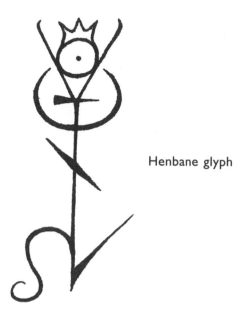

Henbane glyph

are evident due to the discovery of henbane seeds in the burial grounds of the *völva,* the ancient seer-songstresses of the Northern Tradition, the ancient religion of the Germanic and Scandinavian peoples.

This discovery and the subsequent discovery of seeds in other burial sites attests to the long history of the plant's use in shamanic traditions and its connection to the dead. The seeds, flowers, and pods of the plant can be given to the dead as offerings by burying them in a small hole dug by the witch's own hands in a rite of interment. Alternatively, they can be left in graveyards, among animal remains, or in other places where death is present. Henbane is a powerful ally when one is seeking the aid of spirits and can be taken to graveyards, crossroads, and other wayside places where the plant likes to grow. The physical appearance of this plant is otherworldly; the pale flowers with their dark reddish-purple veins and seedpods shaped like cauldrons or funerary vessels are sympathetic to this plant's magic. The plant can be used to adorn ancestral altars, in Samhain rites, and to conceal one's working from others under its Saturnian influence.

As a necromantic tool, henbane seeds offer the sorcerer an experience that is similar in effect to that of other solanaceous plants, being slightly safer and more predictable than henbane's sister *Atropa belladonna*. The trance that henbane induces comes on more subtly and is not as harsh as that of belladonna, which can quickly take on a life of its own. The henbane trance has more of a warming, floating quality to it, with strong soporific effects. While henbane is still a deadly poison, its spirit seems less sadistic than deadly nightshade. Burning henbane should be done outdoors or in a well-ventilated area where excess smoke can escape after the initial inhalation, rising to meet the spirits. Henbane produces numerous tiny seeds, which coincide with Mercurian herbs. A small pinch of fifteen to twenty seeds is enough to produce enough smoke to be effective without overwhelming the senses, but it is always a good idea to start with a smaller amount and determine how everyone responds.

Henbane acts as a guide, allowing us to travel to the spirit world through visionary means, retrieving information that would otherwise be forgotten. The seductive qualities of the plant can be used in spells of coercion and amorous manipulation, dulling the senses and inspiring lust. They can be used to magically lull an enemy into a sense of complacency to divulge secrets or allow one to cross an enemy's barriers without notice. Henbane oil has also been employed as an erotic massage oil for its aphrodisiac properties with warming and relaxing effects. It can also be dried and included in poppets used in dark love spells when combined with Venusian herbs.

Henbane Dosages and Preparation

The lethal dosage of henbane is unknown. It is one of the milder nightshades and a safe one to start with. There are no deaths that have been irrefutably linked to the use of henbane. Young leaves and stems can be used for the expression of juice, while a plaster or poultice of dried leaves is ideal for relieving pain such as rheumatism and neuralgia. As a sedative application for rheumatism, a maceration of leaves and alcohol is mixed with olive oil. The oil is heated until the alcohol evaporates, leaving behind the extracted alkaloids. The mature leaves and flowering tops can be collected for tincturing. A vinegar tincture of henbane can be applied to the temples and forehead for headache, fever, and restless sleep. The fumes of burning henbane were traditionally inhaled for the rapid reduction of swelling related to toothache.

Therapeutic applications are typically 0.5 g up to 3 g. The standard alkaloid content is reported to range from 0.03 to 0.28 percent (Rätsch 2005, 281). However, other ranges have also been given, which shows the variations of alkaloid content based on environmental factors. The percentages of alkaloids of henbane are 0.17 percent (leaves), 0.08 percent (roots), and 0.05 percent (seeds) (Grieve 1971; Frohne and Pfander 1983, cited in Alizadeh et al. 2014; Begum 2010, cited in Alizadeh et al. 2014). While the findings of alkaloid content from various sources are sometimes contradictory, it is known that Egyptian henbane (*H muticus*) has a higher alkaloid content than *H. niger*, which is 0.7 to 1.5 percent by weight (Alizadeh et al. 2014).

⁂

Bilsenkraut Beer

Henbane, called Bilsenkraut *in German, was once added to beer to increase its intoxicating effects by compounding the effects of the alcohol. Henbane beer makes a great ritual beverage that can be enjoyed on special occasions.*

- 40 g henbane, dried and chopped
- 5 g bayberry (optional)
- 25 liters water
- 1 liter brewing malt
- 900 g honey
- 5 g dried yeast
- Brown sugar

Put the henbane and bayberry (if included) in one liter of water and bring to a boil to sterilize; leave to cool. Sterilize a brewing vessel, which can be a plastic bucket with a lid, by rinsing it with boiling water. After rinsing, add and dissolve the liquid malt and honey in two liters of hot water. Add the henbane water, including the herbage, and stir thoroughly. Add enough cold water to make approximately 25 liters of liquid. Add the yeast and cover. Allow it to stand at a temperature of 68–77 degrees Fahrenheit, an optimum temperature for promoting yeast fermentation. Due to the presence of tropane alkaloids, fermentation is slower, the majority occurring in four to five days. Once the yeast begins to settle to the bottom, the beer can be bottled. A teaspoon of brown sugar can be added to each bottle to promote additional fermentation. This beer is best after being stored in a cool, dark place for two to three months (Rätsch 2005, 279).

ॐ

Ritual Fumigant to Conjure and See Spirits

- 🌢 4 parts henbane (*Hyoscyamus niger*) seeds
- 🌢 1 part cassia (*Cinnamomum cassia*) bark
- 🌢 1 part coriander (*Coriandrum sativum*) seeds
- 🌢 1 part fennel (*Foeniculum vulgare*) roots and seeds
- 🌢 1 part olibanum/frankincense (*Boswellia sacra*)

The sorcerer would take this mixture to a forest late at night, when the spirits manifest themselves. The sorcerer would burn the blend on a tree stump alongside a black candle until the candle went out (Hylsop and Ratcliffe 1989, cited in Rätsch 2005, 281).

Burn this blend to aid in the manifestation of spirits and to contact the dead. Be cautious of how much you are burning, especially if you are doing it indoors. Add just a small pinch at a time and observe the effects.

ॐ

Henbane Tincture (Church and Church 2009)

- 🌢 1 part *Hyoscyamus niger* leaves and flowers
- 🌢 10 parts 70 percent alcohol

Harvest the leaves and flowers in June, before plant goes to seed. Shred or chop the plant material and macerate in alcohol for ten to fourteen days. Dose is 5–10 ml per week.

Poison Hemlock (*Conium maculatum*): The Mark of Cain

Hemlock is a poisonous plant that has been used since antiquity. Surprisingly, it does not get the attention that other herbs connected to witches and sorcery, like the nightshade family, do. It is one of the most common plants associated with witches in Europe, particularly in Britain, one of the plant's native homes. Like many of the baneful herbs, hemlock is connected to Hecate and Saturnus. It was also used by the infamous sorceresses Circe and Medea to dispatch many of their male enemies. This also relates to the plant's ability to destroy male potency, virility, and sexual drive. It is used in folk magic to ruin sexual urges and in spells of chastity.

Magically, poison hemlock can be used to paralyze a person or situation, which corresponds to its chemical action on the nervous system. The plant causes death through respiratory failure and acts on the peripheral nervous system, causing coldness, depression, paralysis, and weakness. It is involved in astral travel, like other plants that loosen the soul from the body. As a powerful herb of consecration and protection, it can be used in oils to anoint ritual tools and destructive charms. Hemlock has an earthy and watery nature based on its large chambered root and affinity for growing near streams.

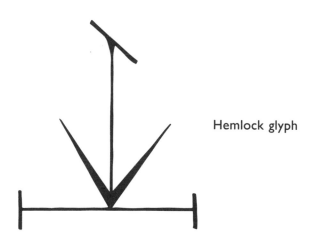

Hemlock glyph

Some of poison hemlock's folk names are warlock's weed, winter fern, poison parsley, and water parsley. The variety native to Europe, *Conium maculatum,* was originally referred to in folklore as witches' weed. *Conium* comes from the Greek word *konas,* meaning "to spin" or "to whirl," likely from the vertigo caused when the plant is consumed. It causes a feeling of dizziness and movement, even when sitting still. When taken in small amounts or rubbed on the skin, this dangerous plant is said to give one the sensation of gliding through the air. This may be why it is connected to witches' flying ointments in medieval Europe. Poison hemlock can be distinguished from other varieties sharing the same common name by the delicate serration in its leaves, as well as the purple spotting that is characteristic of this variety, appropriately known as the mark of Cain.

It is said that ancient Sumerians used the plant to bring about plagues and pestilence and conversely to expel them. Its suffocating side effects connect it to the noose and the dark goddess in her "strangler" aspect—an ancient translation associated with Lilith and the dark goddess Kali.

A genus related to *Conium* is *Cicuta,* which has several varieties common in North America. These two genera are part of the same family, which goes by two different names: Apiaceae and Umbelliferae. Umbelliferae refers to the plant's umbrella-like flowers, called umbels. The *Cicuta* genus is a small group with varieties known as water hemlock (*Cicuta douglasii*), cowbane (*Cicuta virosa*), and spotted cowbane (*Cicuta maculata*). All these plants are widely naturalized outside their native origins, although remaining in the Northern Hemisphere. Typically, only *Conium maculatum* has the purple spotting, but it has been known to show up on other varieties as well, such as *Cicuta maculata*. *Cicuta* varieties commonly grow near streams, along trails and roadsides, and in forest clearings. It is a genus of borders, wastelands, and in-between areas, a typical characteristic of plants used in spirit flight.

The two genera *Cicuta* and *Conium* were not distinguished from one another until after the year 1500. The difference can be seen in the shape of their leaves. The leaves in the *Cicuta* variety are lanceolate and serrate. You can also see characteristic purple coloring at the junctions between branches. Water hemlock is considered one of North America's most toxic plants. It has been confused with wild parsnip and carrot and is similarly related to angelica.

All varieties of *Cicuta* but one contain cicutoxins, which are present during all stages of growth and are particularly concentrated in the roots. It takes only a small amount of the plant to cause lethal poisoning. There have been reports of children poisoned by whistles made from the hollow stems of the plant. Toxicity sets in quickly, just fifteen minutes following ingestion. The poison causes neurological symptoms, including, seizures, hallucinations, brain swelling, delirium, prickling, and numbness. Initial treatment can include the use of activated charcoal to decontaminate the gastrointestinal tract. There is no specific antidote for water hemlock poisoning aside from supportive care, including the use of antiseizure medications.

The primary toxin in *Conium maculatum* is coniine, which is similar in chemical structure to nicotine. It is a piperidine alkaloid, which disrupts the activity of the central nervous system, causing muscular weakness and respiratory paralysis. The ripe seeds contain the most concentrated presence of the poison, and only a very small amount can cause respiratory failure and death. Coniine is unstable, and the dried plant material quickly loses its toxicity in a couple of days. The process of coniine poisoning results in ascending muscular paralysis, starting at the lower extremities and rising to the heart and lungs. It takes as few as six leaves to cause death in adults and even smaller amounts of the seeds. Unlike other neurotoxins, it does not cause intense pain, convulsions, or disorientation and was likely thought of as a more humane means of execution in the ancient world. Some animals that feed on the plant can develop chronic toxicity, which results in birth defects. It is also capable of entering the human food chain through contaminated milk and poultry.

It is no wonder that there are only small amounts of lore that can be found on this plant for magical uses. Other than its association with witches and the devil, uses of this poisonous plant are few and far between. It is a plant that warrants further exploration; however, the utmost precautions must be taken when working directly with either *Cicuta* or *Conium* species.

Anointing Magical Weapons with Hemlock

Hemlock can be used to consecrate and empower ritual tools such as a sword, sickle, athame (black-handled double-edged dagger), or boline (white-handled ritual knife). A water-based infusion or a ritual oil can be made using a small amount of dried hemlock. Avoid using fresh plant material because it is more toxic. If you are using the water infusion, you can heat the blade in the flame of a candle and plunge it into the liquid to help fuse the vibrations. An anointing oil can be used in a similar manner by applying it from the tip of the blade to the base of the handle. If the handle is wooden, it can also be applied there. To make the liquid, add a pinch of plant material to a bowl of water, place on an altar or outdoors, and let their vibrations mingle overnight.

☙

Black Hellebore (*Helleborus niger*):
A Cure for Madness

The *Helleborus* genus has many varieties and hybrid species, and like the other infamous herbs of the Poison Path, it has an extensive history in medicine and magic. Mention of this plant goes all the way back to ancient Greece, and it is said to have been a common prescription of Hippocrates for insanity and mania. In the Greek language, its name refers directly to its poisonous nature (*helein,* "to kill," and *bora,* "food"). It is found in Faustian rituals of exorcism and the coercion of spirits and also mentioned by both Pliny the Elder and the German physician Heinrich Cornelius Agrippa (1486–1535).

It is a member of the Ranunculaceae family, the buttercups, which are all generally poisonous to one degree or another. The toxin within the plant is helleborin, which gives the plant its burning acrid taste.

The horrible taste makes it difficult for one to unintentionally consume enough of the plant for it to be lethal, usually resulting in it being spit out before its intense purgative effects set in. Helleborcin is another toxin within the plant that has a sweet sort of taste, acting in a similar way to the highly active cardiac poisons found in *Digitalis* (foxglove).

Poisoning by this plant causes tinnitus, vertigo, stupor, and thirst. It also includes a feeling of suffocation and swelling of the tongue and throat, followed by violent emesis (vomiting) and a slowing of the heart rate until it causes death by cardiac arrest. It will also burn the eyes and irritate the skin when in direct content with the juice of the plant, including contact with bruised leaves. Chemically, its constituents are related to the venom found in certain toad skin.

As with many of the most well-known plants of the witch's garden, hellebore has a dark and otherworldly beauty. The varied colors of its unique flowers are deep violets, dark reddish pink, and pale green to white. The long-lasting flowers have a more leaflike appearance than that of a delicate flower petal. The seeds are difficult to germinate, but once established the plant cares for itself. For this reason, it was traditionally planted above graves in Europe. The petals catch the moonlight, giving them a ghostly glow. The plant oftentimes does not bloom until its third year, but it is one of the earliest blooming flowers. Blooming between December and February, hellebore was named Christmas or Lenten rose.

In Christian plant lore, this dark herb was ironically seen as a symbol of innocence. It was considered holy and able to ward off evil spirits. According to Christian mythology, the Christmas rose grew from the tears of an empty-handed girl in the presence of the Christ child, for whom she had no gift.

In medieval esoteric and occult lore, we find the more magically appropriate astrological associations applied to this plant. These connections more closely represent its uses and myths from the ancient world.

In ancient Greece, hellebore was called *melampodium,* after the physician and soothsayer Melampus, who used it to cure King Proetus's three daughters of madness. According to one version of the myth, they did not accept the new rites of Dionysus and so he drove them into madness, much like the maenads who worshipped him. The much-feared maenads were female worshippers known for the ecstatic frenzies they would achieve.

As one of the classical witchcraft herbs of medieval lore, *Helleborus niger* has associations with necromancy, the dark goddess, raising and banishing spirits, and appeasing spiritual forces when they have been disturbed. Black hellebore also has a connection to elemental water and its subterranean qualities, and it acts as a portal to the otherworld, subconscious, and lower realms.

In medieval medicine, it was used to cure demonic possession, madness, and epilepsy. At that time, these conditions would have been seen as one ailment. The powdered roots and leaves would be smoldered to calm one already in a frenzy. Hellebore had a reputation for its connection to madness and mental deterioration, creating a catatonic-like state in those suffering the madness of maenads; however, in healthy individuals, it would induce similar symptoms, which speak to its homeopathic uses. The idea is that in small amounts homeopathic remedies would cure the symptoms that in large amounts it would cause. It has been used in curses of insanity and held as the antidote for its cure.

Hellebore glyph

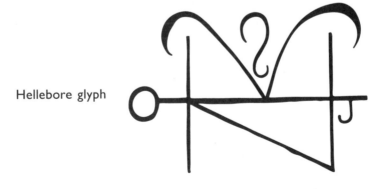

Hellebore in Magical Practice

One of the more interesting magical uses mentioned is that hellebore would be used to alter or change the nature of another plant either through grafting living hellebore to that plant or by powdering it and using it as a fertilizer. Through magical transference, it was said to give the plant and its fruits unpleasant and unhealthy qualities. This would make it a useful herb in charms of blighting to curse a piece of land, which was often a popular accusation during the witch craze in Europe.

An interesting piece of French lore, mentioned by author, folklorist, and herbalist Maud Grieve, concerns a sorcerer who used its powers of invisibility to move about unseen through enemy lines by throwing the powdered plant in the air about himself. The plant has also been used in rites of exorcism, banishment, and protection. It can be applied in curse work and spells of revenge. In addition to its powers of altering perception, it is connected to rebirth and gaining intelligence through spiritual means. If there were one poisonous plant that most closely reflected the nature of the medieval magician and his machinations, it would be *Helleborus niger*. Just as deadly nightshade has connections with the witches of medieval folklore, black hellebore seems to be the perfect male counterpart.

In Agrippa's *Three Books of Occult Philosophy,* he places black hellebore under the rulership of Mars and Saturn, suggesting its use in the fumigation of talismans of the same correspondence. In medieval astrology, the legendary Hermes Trismegistus associates the plant with the demon star Algol. Well known for its malefic attributions, this star is found in the constellation of Perseus representing the head of the slain Medusa. According to medieval hermetic manuscripts, the juice of black hellebore and wormwood, placed under a diamond and under the influence of this fixed star, would bring about hatred and courage as well as protection and preservation of the body, and it would bring vengeance to all one's enemies. As an amulet of protection, the black roots of *H. niger* can be prepared and carried like a mandragora.

This beautiful plant is still popular in rustic gardens and medieval apothecaries. It brings otherworldly beauty to the otherwise frozen skeleton of the winter garden. The wide varieties of *Helleborus* come in many colors. There are many people who grow it as a hobby plant, for its unique beauty. This woodland herb stands in stark contrast to the muted colors of late winter.

THE ARTEMISIAS: MUGWORT AND WORMWOOD

These two plants, mugwort and wormwood, are in the *Artemisia* genus, which is named after the Greek goddess Artemis (Diana in Roman mythology). They are staples in any witch's herb cabinet and are classic herbs of witchery. They are traditionally known for their powers of magical enhancement, spirit work, and divination. The plants are frequently used together as they complement one another, with mugwort being feminine and wormwood masculine. They are used in incense to induce a trance and aid divination and as spirit offerings when performing ritual. Easy to grow and safe to use, mugwort and wormwood are made into oils for anointing ritual tools, especially those used for divination. Lustral waters can be made from these plants through infusion and used to consecrate and bless sacred spaces or poured in libations to deities.

🌱

Mugwort (*Artemisia vulgaris*): Protector and Diviner

Mugwort is a feminine herb intimately connected to the moon and sacred to goddesses that rule the lunar sphere, and it can be used to connect with dark moon and crone goddesses. It can be used to heal traumas to the *anima,* the sacred feminine within all of us. Mugwort is used in traditional Chinese medicine to restore yin deficiencies, balancing the masculine and feminine chi within a person.

It has been known by other names, such as cronewort, felon herb, and the Old English *yldost wyrta,* which means "oldest wort." In Anglo-Saxon lore it was known as one of the nine sacred healing herbs of the famed Nine Herbs Prayer. The recipe for this medical prescription was recorded in the *Lacnunga* ("Remedies"), a collection of Anglo-Saxon prayers and remedies, and it was said to have many magical properties. Some of its properties are protection, strength, psychic communication, prophetic dreaming, healing, and astral projection.

Mugwort is one of the primary divinatory herbs used to enhance psychic ability, aid in rituals of prophecy, and promote prophetic dreams. Like wormwood, it contains the alkaloid thujone. It can be burned as a fumigant in scrying rituals to alter consciousness and for the same purpose can be taken as a tea sweetened with honey. When burned as an incense, mugwort is commonly mixed with wormwood and sandalwood. When made into an infusion or wash, the herb can be used to sprinkle on the altar or table where divination is performed.

An infusion of mugwort can also be used to wash scrying mirrors, attune pendulums, and charge runes or cards. Her feminine lunar energy infuses these tools with the proper vibrations to enhance their effectiveness. Mugwort is a well-known dreaming herb and can be drunk as a tea before bed to enhance dream recall. It is also used in dream magic as a dream pillow, added to sachets of dreaming herbs and placed under the pillow. The essential oil of mugwort may also be used to enhance dreaming by being placed in a diffuser near the bed or applied with carrier oil beneath the nose so its scent can be inhaled throughout the night; the latter has a more potent effect than the former. Mugwort essential oil should not be ingested internally.

The plant can be used as a smudge for cleansing rituals of both people and places. It is often incorporated into smudge bundles used for purification and burned as an incense for the same. Native Americans use mugwort to rid people of ghosts by burning the plant or rubbing it on the skin of the afflicted.

Medicinally, it has been used in the Eastern practice of *moxibustion,* where plant material is ignited on the surface of the skin to increase circulation and reduce pain and irritation over joints and muscles. It is used to treat digestive issues and parasitic infections as it has antibacterial and antifungal properties. As a women's health herb, mugwort was traditionally taken to regulate menstruation and as such may have been used as an abortifacient. For this reason, mugwort should not be taken by women who are pregnant or who seek to conceive.

It has been used to treat nervousness, exhaustion, and depression and is said to have mild narcotic and sedative properties. Both the aerial parts of the plant and the roots may be used. Mugwort contains beneficial volatile oils and triterpenes.

Mugwort Dosages and Preparation

Mugwort can be taken internally as a tea or an extract to produce relaxation and clear the mind. Smoking mugwort, drinking tea, or taking a tincture or extract intensifies dream clarity and recall.

Essential oil: Use mugwort essential oil on a dream pillow or apply to the third eye and temples to access intuition.

Infusion: One to two teaspoons of dried herb to one cup of boiling water; infuse for ten to fifteen minutes in a covered container. Drink prior to divination or before sleeping to dream of an answer to a question.

Tincture: Take a few drops of mugwort tincture in a cup of chamomile tea before bed to encourage vivid dreams.

Smoking blend: The dried plant may be smoked alone or in a blend. Use one to three grams for psychoactive effects, such as mild and pleasant stimulation and increased euphoria.

꙳

Wormwood (Artemisia absinthium): The Wild Green Man

Wormwood complements the feminine nature of mugwort. It is a masculine spirit that is fiery and trickster-like, appearing as a devilish green man. It is burned to call upon spirits of the dead and can be used for purification in necromantic rituals without clearing away spirits. In the Northern Tradition, wormwood is sacred to Hel and her underworld guardian Mordgud. Wormwood can be used to petition this gatekeeper to enter Elivdnir, Hel's Hall. It can aid in rituals meant to release the wandering dead and send them to Helheim (House of Hell).

Like the other *Artemisia* species, it is sacred to the goddess Artemis-Diana and other lunar deities, including Hecate, and can be taken as a sacrament during full moon rituals to symbolically ingest these goddesses (Rätsch 2005). In addition to lunar goddesses, wormwood is also favored by the goddess Lilith. It is said to have sprouted from the ground in the wake of the serpent as it was exiled from the Garden of Eden. In the Book of Revelation, wormwood is the name of a star or possibly an angel that is one of the harbingers of Armageddon.

> *The third angel sounded his trumpet, and a great star, blazing like a torch, fell from the sky on a third of the rivers and on the springs of water—the name of the star is Wormwood. A third of the waters turned bitter, and many people died from the waters that had become bitter.*
>
> REVELATION 8:10–11

Magically, wormwood can be used for psychic work, protection, and calling spirits. It is a powerful banishing herb that purges parasitic entities and clears the energy field. As a ritual incense, it can be used in Samhain rites for evocation and divination. In addition to its lunar affinity as an *Artemisia* species, wormwood is ruled by Mars and Pluto. Culpeper associated wormwood with Mars because of its warming properties. It was suggested as a remedy for the stings of Martian creatures like scorpions, wasps, and snakes.

An effective ingredient in spells of vengeance, wormwood can be used to stop conflict by inhibiting the enemy or in return-to-sender spells to seal negativity with its source. Steeping wormwood in magical ink will protect what is written through sympathetic magic. As a vermicide, it was used as a strewing herb and as an additive to ink to protect pages from mice.

Wormwood contains the volatile oil thujone, a monoterpene. Like other *Artemisia* species, in tincture form it can be mildly psychoactive. The leaves near the flowering tops are thought to contain higher amounts of the alkaloid (Rätsch 2005, 71–72).

Wormwood Dosages and Preparation

The dried herb can be smoked alone or in a smoking blend. Burning it as an incense with camphor increases its psychoactive effects through chemical synergy, a combination used in the *Grande Grimoire*.

As a bitter tea, 0.5 to 1 g of leaves in one cup of boiling water is considered a medicinal dose. Wormwood is known for its bitter taste and can be mixed with sweeter herbs or honey in tea. Like mugwort, wormwood should be avoided by pregnant women. It is an abortifacient and was used in traditional herbal preparations to induce menstruation and induce labor.

༺༻

Artemisia Tea

- 🌿 1 Tbsp. wormwood
- 🌿 1 Tbsp. mugwort
- 🌿 2–3 star anise pods

Infuse the herbs in one cup of hot water for fifteen minutes. Drink this tea thirty minutes prior to any psychic working. The tea helps lower inhibitions and focus the mind to access intuition more easily. It is especially effective in scrying and dream divination, which relies on images coming into the conscious mind. It is also a good tonic before rituals involving the moon because of the herbs' lunar associations. Use it to draw down lunar energy for spell work and to connect with lunar deities.

Caution: Don't drink this tea if you are pregnant or trying to become pregnant.

༃

Agrimony (*Agrimonia eupatoria*): Protector of Witches

Boundaries, containment, and division are all Saturnian qualities. Like the rings that surround the planet itself, the magical circle is both a protective boundary and a container for the energies raised within. The circle divides the mundane world from the spiritual reality created within.

Agrimony, according to medieval lore, has a Jupiterian and masculine energy, being one of the foremost plants of protection against witchcraft. Although magical practitioners describe the spirit of this plant as feminine in form, it has a strong and defensive personality. The Jovian god of the sky rules the many-flowered portion of the plant above, while its dark and woody root belies a more Saturnian nature beneath the surface. The god of thunder offers the more offensive protection of a warrior, while the dark spirit of the root conveys a subtler aspect of protection beneath the surface.

This plant is an ally to those who specialize in defensive magic and helping those who are under psychic attack. It can be especially beneficial to those practitioners who are more public and can be susceptible to regular energetic intrusions and attacks. Agrimony is quick to come to the aid of those who call upon it and is especially potent when it comes to combating harmful magic that has already been put into motion. The powdered root can be used to erect powerful protective wards.

Agrimony was used by the Anglo-Saxons to stop bleeding and heal wounds, a practical application for those in battle. This connection to healing the flesh, the protective tissue, translates to the energy body as well. It can be employed to heal the anatomy of the aura when it is damaged after a traumatic experience and for the removal of attachments. It quickly heals the aura and ensures the aura is well fortified against further damage during the healing process.

It can also be used in magical retaliation; when included in protective wards, it not only defends the area but pursues the offenders with a vengeance. The sealing properties of the plant can be used in return-to-sender spells to both return negativity and keep it there.

In addition to its protective capabilities, the lore of this plant mentions its peculiar reputation for causing sleep when placed under a pillow. It can keep someone already sleeping in an unconscious state until the plant is removed. In the past, witches did this to their sleeping spouses, enabling them to secretly attend the witches' sabbat—an interesting effect warranting further experimentation. Since the herb itself is non-narcotic, its soporific action is achieved by more occult means.

✹

Solomon's Seal (*Polygonatum odoratum*): The Magical Catalyst

Solomon's seal, named after the magician-king of antiquity to whom many magical acts and texts are attributed, is a potent example of a magical catalyst. It is also a powerful medicinal herb that helps with musculoskeletal issues. Saturn is the ruler of the skeletal system in medical astrology, as well as elemental earth. The root's resemblance to the human spine and its effects on ligaments, tendons, and bones earns it a place in the Book of Saturn. The plant when taken medicinally affects the connective tissues of the human body, allowing them to either contract or relax depending on the issue, which creates a relaxing and pain-relieving effect for issues of the back, joints, and muscles.

This plant is useful in protection spells and works of banishing and exorcisms, for which King Solomon was famous. By binding and exorcising demonic spirits, he was able to construct the sacred Temple of Solomon. Pieces of the root can be placed in the four corners of the home to act as a protective spell to ward off negativity or as a means of containment. When placed purposefully, the roots act to create an etheric structure that is capable of either keeping in what is desired or restricting access to that which is unwanted. The Saturnian influence of this plant makes its especially useful at creating boundaries. Because of its proficiency with binding and crystallization, it is useful for sealing oaths and magical contracts, as well as binding one's magic to the material plane.

When used in a similar way on the human energy field, it helps us adapt to different situations, allowing the aura to tighten or relax depending on the circumstances. The aura can become porous and absorbent, allowing energy to pass through it, or it can harden, creating a protective shell to keep out harmful forces. Solomon's seal can be combined with yarrow and labradorite, a feldspar mineral, in a charm to protect, fortify, and defend the aura. All three ingredients work to strengthen the aura in different ways.

This plant's name evokes an image of a wizard king of old, connecting it to ceremonial magic. It is said to have been used in ancient times to consecrate and empower ritual tools and as a general elemental offering. The plant has six petals, which make the shape of the hexagram, the symbol inscribed on the magical ring of King Solomon.

In occult symbolism, the hexagram represents the microcosm and macrocosm as well as the union between masculine and feminine energies. It also contains the alchemical figures of the four elements. The planetary and elemental forces are also contained in the geometry of the hexagram, representing a gateway.

The root of Solomon's seal can be made into a tincture and taken to imbue the beneficial powers of this plant into one's physical body, thereby allowing one's magical energy to flow more freely, balancing the aura. It can be added to any formula to increase its efficacy, and when paired with other ingredients, it is able to take on and enhance those qualities due to the plant's versatile nature. It can teach the magician much about elemental magic and planetary forces by acting as a plant teacher and familiar spirit. It can assist in the assimilation of new information in the arcane applications of plant magic.

6

The Book of Venus

The Ars Veneris

*V*enus is the goddess of love and beauty, an innocent daughter of the sea. She rules the arts of lovemaking, glamour, and personal beauty. As an emanation of the Great Goddess, she embodies all things feminine and nurturing, but like her male counterparts, she has another side that reveals itself with further investigation. She is closely associated with Mercury, the planet that is closest in orbit to her. They rule over the personal sphere and our relationships with other people. Venus represents the *anima,* the feminine principle within humanity and the individual, while Mercury represents the *animus,* the masculine principle. They are two parts of a whole, a fully realized individual represented by the deity Hermaphrodite, who combines the female and male aspects of Aphrodite and Hermes. They represent a sacred union, the *hieros gamos,* an alchemical transformation. Venus is not without her masculine qualities, as Mercury also has his feminine side.

Venus and Mercury are located between Earth and the sun, giving them the positioning to rise before the sun during part of the year and follow it as it sets during the rest. This rising and setting with the sun make both planets light bringers and night bringers, which speaks of their dual nature. As Phosphoros, Venus is the Morning Star, bringing the light of illumination through the celestial spheres, seen as a rainbow of colors, which are the emanations of the moon, a reflection of the influence of all the planetary bodies and fixed stars. As Hesperos or Noctifer, she is the Evening Star, bringing darkness and shadow over

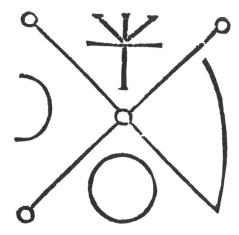

Planetary seal of Venus
(From Agrippa, *Three Books of Occult Philosophy*)

the world. She is the Witch Star or the Queen of the Sabbath, bringing with her the mysteries of the world of shadow.

The astrological glyph of Venus is the circle of the soul above the elemental cross of matter (see the upper left corner of the triangle on page 38). It reminds us that the cosmic laws of the celestial spheres above are mirrored in the laws of nature below. Venus is the manifestation of these cosmic forces in the natural world. She is the goddess of the plant realm and the bounty of nature. Her glyph also represents the looking glass, which symbolizes not only the physical beauty of the reflection but also the reflective nature of the moon. This is the hidden world beyond the veil, the subconscious and the deep dark waters of the underworld. By descending to the depths of the well, the darkest parts of ourselves, we reach the part of us connected to the all. The primordial waters of creation teach us through vision and dream that the material world reflects the spiritual world, and after our journey to the depths, we return to the surface with this wisdom.

Astrologically, Venus rules the signs of Taurus and Libra. The second house, ruled by Taurus, is the house of possessions, not only material possessions but the natural talents we possess as well. It represents our available resources and how we can use them to our best advantage.

The seventh house ruled by Libra is the house of partnerships,

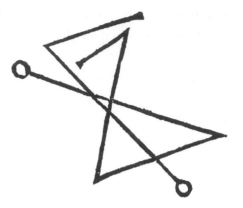

Sigil of the intelligence of Venus
(From Agrippa, *Three Books
of Occult Philosophy*)

romantic relationships, and spiritual interactions. It teaches us how to balance such relationships. It is the house of channeling and communication with the divine as much as it is our relationships with our fellow humans; it teaches us how we view ourselves and the role that we play by reflecting to us what we see in the mirror.

Astrologers call Venus the "lesser fortunate," as she is the lower octave of Jupiter, the "greater fortunate." Both planets are known for bestowing their blessings upon Earth, and this correspondence is reflected in their position on the Tree of Life. Chokmah, ruled by Jupiter, is the higher sphere above Netzach, the sphere of Venus. Her negative aspects are jealousy, vanity, and narcissism. In Greek mythology, Aphrodite was known for her jealously and pride, as much as she was for her beauty. Although she is the mirror opposite of Mars, the god of war, she was often caught up in quarrels between the gods and was the impetus for wars among the ancients. Each part is said to contain its opposite; that is the nature of things, and the gods are no exception.

Like the Great Mother who nurtures and protects her children, Venus can also be destructive and chaotic. The void from which all potential arises contains all opposites, both dark and light. The cycle of life and death is intimately connected to and embodied by the Great Goddess. Sex and death are both represented by the zodiac sign Scorpio, the sign in opposition to Taurus. The primordial waters that we emerge from at birth are the same as the waters that flow through the rivers we cross in death. The forces of life and death are inextricably connected with the concept of fate or destiny, the inescapable wheel of incarnation.

Venus presides over the craft of the herbalist and wort cunner. She is the queen in the garden, depicted on the empress card in the tarot. She is present in the Garden of the Hesperides, the Garden of Eden, and the shadow garden of Hecate. Her waters of transmutation, which fill the cauldron, are the basis for making potions of balm or bane. The five-petaled flowers that correspond to her nature are gateway plants that are, on the one hand, miraculous healers and, on the other, swift poisons. They are plants that bring great relief, allowing the life force to flow uninhibited, and venefic herbs that draw the vital force out. These are the great witching herbs; when employed by those who know their mysteries, they can help us reach the space between life and death. They help us achieve spirit flight and act as profound teachers.

22	47	16	41	10	35	4
5	23	48	17	42	11	29
30	6	24	49	18	36	12
13	31	7	25	43	19	37
38	14	32	1	26	44	20
21	39	8	33	2	27	45
46	15	40	9	34	3	28

Kamea of Venus
(From Agrippa, *Three Books of Occult Philosophy*)

Herbs of glamour and enchantment are under Venus's domain as well. The soothing, astringent, and tonic herbs used for lustral waters of beautification, maintaining youth, and imparting otherworldly allure have been the secret of cunning women passed on through the ages. Many of these plants continue to be used as ingredients in modern cosmetics. In addition to enhancing and maintaining natural beauty, many of these plants have been used to create illusions and charms of enchantment. Aphrodisiacs used to inspire lust and dull the senses have been used to enhance virility and amorousness and ensnare the senses of a would-be suitor. These are known as the ars Veneris, the art of Venus or venereal arts, capable of lighting the fires of passion and also snuffing them out. Aphrodisiacs and anaphrodisiacs were part of the repertoire of infamous witches of old.

FREYA: BATTLE, SORCERY, AND LOVE

In the Northern Tradition of the Norse and Germanic peoples, the goddess Freya is the most closely aligned with Venus. The deities of the Northern Tradition are more ambiguous, with a wide range of overlapping attributes. Their dark and light halves are more clearly manifested, and the division between one goddess or spirit and another is not always clearly defined. Freya is the goddess of love, fertility, beauty, and material possessions. She is known for being passionate about the pleasures of this world. Freya is also depicted as a fierce and powerful goddess of warfare and sorcery. Her powers are unrivaled, like those of the Fates. She can manipulate the desires as well as the health and prosperity of others. She can discern the currents of *wyrd* through *seidr,* a type of Norse witchcraft that works through divination. The Northern Tradition concept of wyrd roughly corresponds to fate or personal destiny. By divining the wyrd or fate of others, Freya can manipulate the outcomes.

She is the first and archetypal völva or seeress. She is credited with teaching Odin the practice of seidr, traditionally practiced by females. This was a combination of sorcery and shamanism, in which the practitioner would create change by altering the structures of fate itself. The term *völva,* used to describe these traveling seeresses who practiced magic, is similar in meaning to *witch.*

Freya is also a shape-shifter who uses enchanted falcon feathers to transform herself into this bird of war. Her connection to the battlefield can be seen through the role of the *veleda.* An integral part of the traveling warband in Norse and Germanic tribal cultures, the veleda was the wife of the chieftain who led the warband, and she played a pivotal role in divining the outcomes of battle and used her magic to sway the tides of war. Freya is synonymously linked with Frigg, the wife of Odin, who fulfilled a similar role in the battles between Aesir and Vanir. Freya was a member of the Vanir tribe of gods but also held honorary status among the Aesir.

Although part of the Norse pantheon, Freya seems to be in a category all her own. A powerful force in her own right, like the Titaness Hecate, Freya presides over her own realm in the Norse afterlife known as Folkvangir, where half of the warriors slain in battle are chosen to go. The other half go with Odin to Valhalla. Like the Fates or Norns, who decide one's destiny and when it is time to die, Freya chooses which of the slain will accompany her in the afterlife.

In the northern Germanic traditions, Freya is often associated with Frau Holt or Holda, who also has connections to Hel, the goddess of the Norse underworld. Holda is known as the Dame of Venus Mountain, which is the site of the witches' sabbat in Germanic lore. Helvegen, the Way to Hell, also known as Venus Road, is at the bottom of the world tree and links to all of the other nine realms. By traveling on Helvegen, via spirit flight and shamanic trance, one can access the power held within the mountain (Frisvold 2014, 77). Mother Holle or Hulda (alternate spellings) has a connection with Lilith as a nocturnal demoness who attacks infants. She is also transformed into the goddess Venus.

THE INEVITABLE POWER OF FATE

The Norns, who are the personifications of the Fates in the Northern Tradition, are known to live at the base of Yggdrasil, the world tree. They dwell within the Well of Urd, also called the Well of Wyrd, and influence the destiny (*wyrd*) of all other beings. The powers of fate play an important role in ancient mythology. To the Greeks they are known as the Moirai, and to the Romans they are the Parcae. It is interesting to note that all of these cultures viewed these primal powers as female personifications. Women held the power of life and death in their hands because it was through them that all humans passed into this world.

In the Northern Tradition the concept of fate was more fluid and alterable. It could be changed through an understanding of the currents of destiny, and through changing one's personal luck through the aid of one's *hamingja*. The hamingja was a kind of guardian spirit that was exclusively female and decided the luck and happiness of the individual, thereby affecting their *wyrd*. The Norns shaped fate by carving runes into the trunk of the world tree and through the art of weaving. In this respect, they are like the magical practitioner, influencing the events around them by working with forces in their environment.

The word *norn,* when written with a lowercase *n,* refers to a general magical practitioner, and in the younger sagas of the Norse, the norns are synonymous with the völva, sorceresses appearing at the birth of a hero to shape his destiny. These female spirits presiding over the destiny of an individual were collectively known as *dísir.* In the Northern Tradition, there are many names for similar spirits that seem to blend together and overlap. These enigmatic female spirits were portrayed as tutelary spirits, acting as guardians of a specific person, family, or location. These spirits were sometimes thought to be the spirits of female ancestors, who were celebrated in the winter at various times by Norse and Germanic peoples. The ritual known as Dísablot was held in honor of these spirits.

The *matres* or *matrones* (Latin words meaning "mothers" or "matrons") of Celtic cultures were also possibly connected with the norns as these female spirits also came in groups of three. These female spirits held a variety of functions as guardians of the land, warrior goddesses, and fertility goddesses. Feasts held in honor of these spirits began in January and were held through February.

The Moirai, like the Norns, belonged to the underworld, secretly guiding the fates of those above. The Three Fates, or Moirai, are descended from Proto-Indo-European cultures. Their origins and actions are shrouded in mystery. In Hesiod's *Theogony,* it is said that the Moirai are the daughters of the primeval goddess of night, Nyx. They are the sisters of her other children Thanatos (death), Nemesis (retribution), and the Keres (black fates). According to Herodotus, the gods themselves are subject to Fates. The Pythian priestess at Delphi said that Zeus is also bound to their powers.

The Moirai or "apportioners" were incarnations of destiny itself. *Moira* or fate (alternately *aisa,* meaning "necessity") was originally a living power related to the limit or end of life, a singular impersonal force; this concept eventually evolved to become the Moirai, the three Fates. Moira was also one's portion of destiny. It included the good and the bad in one's life, and it was impossible for anyone to change the proportions that they were given, something that was predetermined by this universal law. This was different from the constantly unfolding nature of wyrd in the Northern Tradition.

The Three Fates were named Clotho, the spinner, who spun the thread of life from her distaff onto her spindle; Lachesis, the allotter or drawer of lots, who used a measuring rod to determine the length of each person's individual thread or the length of their life; and Atropos, the inexorable or inevitable one, who cut the thread marking the end of a person's life and determined the manner of death.

Fate and destiny are intimately tied to witchcraft and magic. Spinning, weaving, and knot magic are some of the most ancient forms of sorcery. Tying knots was sympathetic to the very action of the Fates themselves and was thought to influence the forces of destiny. By weaving spells, the witch is acting in the capacity of the Fates. Some workings flow in accordance with destiny, while others change it and require some great sacrifice. Magic works by weaving together the threads of reality. The twining of threads, or binding, was a magical art used by sorcerers to harm a person or control his or her individual fate.

The baneful herbs of the Poison Path, plants associated with witches, have an intimate connection to the Fates. They can provide great power and insight but also demand a high price. Vervain (*Verbena officinalis*) is considered an herb of the Norns in the Northern Tradition. It is used in divination, helping one to access the knowledge in the Well of Wyrd to understand the fate of a person. Vervain is used to prepare the altar for divination through the casting of runes or other methods of scrying by brushing the surface upon which the working will take place, sprinkling it over the altar, or using an infusion of the plant as the scrying medium.

> *Listen fates, who sit nearest the throne of Zeus, and weave*
> *shuttles of adamant, inescapable devices of councils for*
> *every kind, beyond counting, Aisa, Clotho, Lachesis, fine*
> *armed daughters of Night. Hearken to our prayers, all*
> *terrible goddesses of earth and sky.*
>
> PINDAR, "HYMN TO THE FATES,"
> FROM *FRAGMENTA CHORICA ADESPOTA*

THE ALCHEMY OF VENUS AND THE ANIMA

Jungian psychology speaks of Venus as the anima, the collective image of the woman inside a man, comprised of his female tendencies. The anima is the feminine side of the human psyche, the feminine lunar energy that balances the masculine solar energy in the cosmos. It is receptive, reflective, and deep and emphasizes feelings, emotions, intuition, receptivity, love of oneself, and nature. These forces are also, of course, present in women and are to be nurtured and embraced as part of themselves. The seductress, the warrior, and the witch are primal female powers suppressed by the patriarchy.

As noted earlier, Venus is the central image of the albedo phase. Born from the sea, Aphrodite guides us through the unconscious (the dark waters of the underworld). The alchemist dives into these depths to find the *prima materia,* the alchemical green lion, which dissolves the heavy metals to their purest forms. The dross or illusions and impurities of spirit that cloud consciousness are the useless matter left behind after this process. In this way, Venus helps us integrate the shadow.

Venus or Aphrodite is the quintessential representation of the feminine, and when combined with Mercury, they form the Hermaphroditic androgyny. This is the balance of salt and sulfur sought by alchemists in the sacred marriage of opposites—the transmutation, the reconciliation and integration of light and darkness.

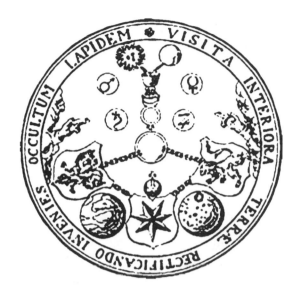

VITRIOL: *Visita Interiora
Terrae Rectificando Invenies
Occultum Lapidem*
(From Basilius Valentinus,
Chymical Wedding,
mid-seventeenth century)

*By her beauty, Venus attracts the imperfect metals and
gives rise to desire and pushes them to perfection and
ripeness.*

Basilius Valentinus, 1679

The female half, assistant, or wife to the alchemist is called the *soror* or *soror mystica,* meaning "mystical sister." The soror represents in part the anima or Venus, as the feminine half of the hiero gamos. Medieval alchemy was dominated by men and alchemical texts were written from a male point of view, but though women's voices were often suppressed, they did practice alchemy. Some of the greatest alchemists were women, and their contributions to the art of fire cannot go unnoticed. For example, the first true alchemist of the Western world was a woman called Miriam the Prophetess. She appeared in the works of Zosimos of Panopolis, a gnostic Christian writer. She was thought to have lived between the first and third centuries CE and is credited with the invention of several alchemical apparatuses.

An Egyptian alchemist who was alive during the first century was rumored to be one of four women who were able to successfully produce the philosopher's stone. In sixteenth- and seventeenth-century France, women both practiced alchemy and advocated for women's rights. Marie Meudrac was a self-taught alchemist who trained other women and wrote a book called *La Chymie Chritable et Facile, en Faveur des Dames* (Useful and Easy Chemistry for the Benefit of Women).

LILITH, THE DARK SIDE OF THE ANIMA

When a woman's primal powers are seen as weaknesses or faults, they are pushed into the subconscious, where they become part of the shadow. This shadow of the feminine side in both males and females is Lilith. Depending on the development of the man, she can manifest as Lilith the dark seductress, luring him away from the Great Work.

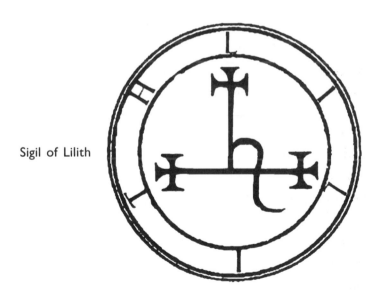

Sigil of Lilith

Lilith is a powerful figure of feminine strength and independence, and because of this she has been demonized for hundreds of years. She represents the wild, seductive, untamed side of feminine nature. She is a deep and dark part of our unconscious, representing our deepest and most secret desires. She is the Great Goddess in her aspect of the destroyer, the devouring mother, known by her epithet "the strangler." She is Lamashtu, a female demon in Mesopotamian mythology, the "darkener of daylight." In ancient Mesopotamia, she is called "the hand of Ishtar."

Lilith is alluded to twice in the Old Testament, first in Genesis and then in Isaiah. There are two versions of the creation myth in Genesis. In one version, man and woman were created at the same time, both from Earth, as equals. The second version says that woman was created from the rib of Adam and was thus a subservient helpmate. In the Book of Genesis 1:27, there is an unnamed allusion to his first wife, who is thought to have been Lilith. The story goes that Lilith, knowing of her equality with Adam, refused to take a submissive position beneath him when they were having sex. Her refusal to submit eventually led to her leaving Adam and fleeing to the Red Sea, where it is said she gave birth to hundreds of demonic offspring fathered by the demon Samael. Lilith and Samael represent the prototypical "unholy pair." They are two of the spheres represented on the Qlipothic Tree of Life. In Jewish mysticism, the Qliphoth, which means "husks" or "shells," respresents evil or impure forces, the opposite of the holy Sephiroth, and displays the destructive side of the divine personality. Lilith is mentioned by name in Isaiah 34:14 as an outcast of the holy land, dwelling with wild cats, hyenas, and goat demons.

Numerous ancient artifacts have been found in connection to Lilith, specifically, in the form of apotropaic charms used to protect against her. She was infamously known for killing infant children in their first few days of life and killing mothers in childbirth. Without modern medicine, numerous complications made infant death a common occurrence in the ancient world. This was a threat to the entire society, and a number of magical precautions were taken to prevent it. There is archaeological evidence of incantation bowls inscribed with charms of protection around their interior, spiraling around images of Lilith. These bowls were buried at the threshold of the front door, with one placed on top of another, creating a spherical container. Several different talismans were also worn or hung in the home with inscriptions of divine and angelic names intended to ward off Lilith's influence. Another interesting type of object used for the same purpose was the talismanic blade, covered in written incantations. One thing is for sure: the presence of Lilith pervaded the ancient world. Considering the importance of perpetuating the survival of these civilizations, their superstitious precautions were a small price to pay to ensure the success of future generations.

Arguably, one of the oldest references to Lilith and figures that contributed to her mythology come from ancient Babylon and Sumer, including the stone inscriptions known as the Burney Relief and the Arslan Tash ivory inscription. They are the oldest depictions of what mythology describes as the characteristics of Lilith. The Burney Relief has possibly the most famous image of Lilith, showing her standing atop two lionesses with two great owls on each side. It also shows her connection to the goddesses Ishtar and Inanna from Babylonian and earlier Sumerian mythology. She appears in the Sumerian poem "Inanna and the Huluppu Tree" and is also mentioned in the Book of Raziel and the Zohar. Parallel myths are seen in ancient Greek mythology in the figure known as Lamia, who played an equally destructive role. Originally, Lamia was a Libyan queen who caught the eye of Zeus. In her jealousy, Hera, the wife of Zeus, cursed Lamia to bring forth only dead children, much like Lilith. In other accounts, Hera murdered Lamia's children, the offspring of Zeus. Out of her despair, Lamia became a demon who kidnaps, strangles, and devours the children of others.

A more contemporary form of Lilith is an amalgam of ancient spirits of the night and the desert, demonic monsters that haunted and seduced the dreams of ancient man. These demons, known as *lilitu* in Jewish mythology, are likely connected to the Assyrian storm demon of the same name. She is a composite of several goddesses and other powerful entities that were transformed by the early patriarchal societies and their religions. Originally, it was the Great Goddess who ruled the magical cycle of life and death, through the powers of sexuality. With the rise of patriarchal society, the power of life and death became the prerogative of the male god, while sexuality and magic were divorced from procreation and motherhood. Lilith stands in opposition to these forms of oppression and teaches us to embrace our desires, go against the norms, and unleash the anima within.

Lilith in Astrology

The biblical telling of the story of Lilith and Adam has parallels in the Hebrew creation myth of the sun and moon in the Book of Genesis. According to the myth, when God created the universe, the sun and the moon were the first two great celestial lights that were created. Neither one of them was willing to share the sky, and in settling this dispute, God sided with the sun, telling the moon to "go and diminish thyself." The moon saw the injustice of losing her own light in deference to the sun and asked, "Why should I be as one who veileth herself?" (Genesis 1:16). This is like Lilith's refusal to submit to Adam. Recognizing her inherent equality, she refused to accept her role.

Astrologically, Lilith is as much of an enigma as her mythological origins. Lilith is the name for three enigmatic astrological phenomena. There is Lilith the asteroid; Dark Moon Lilith, a dust cloud that appears as a kind of ghostly moon, known also as Waldemath's Moon; and Black Moon Lilith, which is not a physical body but a point between the orbit of the moon and Earth. Black Moon Lilith is the second epicenter of the moon's orbit, an invisible point around which the

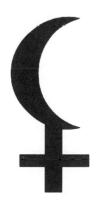

Black Moon Lilith glyph

moon orbits that is closely connected with the center of Earth. It forms an invisible vortex of energy, a place of void. It contains primal energy and potential, manifesting the energy of Earth and sun in the subtle plane. It feeds the subtle currents that flow through Earth, the dark serpent fire that snakes across Earth's surface, manifesting as dragon lines and points of power where they converge.

Lilith is highly individualistic, representing independent and liberated women, as well as men who embrace their primal feminine side. She is a patron of unconventional sexual norms and gender fluidity. She helps us find our personal power and detach ourselves from those who would force us into their conceptions of who we should be.

The nocturnal creatures—owl, wolf, serpent, and moth—all fall under the realm of Lilith. Mythical creatures of the night, such as vampires, werewolves, shape-shifters, and cunning beasts, are also part of her domain. Lilith can teach us to be patient and resourceful, using all of our skills, including aspects of ourselves that we are taught to see as faults, to our advantage. She is a patron of witches and fallen angels, being mother to thousands of children, the children of Cain, those marked as other.

LOVE MAGIC

The arts of making potions, specifically love potions and charms of seduction, fall in the realm of Venus, for which they are named. The *ars Veneris,* as they were once known, were considered a type of malefic magic, occult poisoning of the body and mind of another to seduce him or her. In ancient Rome, poisoning was a crime that was all too common. It was known as *veneficia* or *veneficium* and was synonymous with magic and sorcery. The words *veneficus* (male) or *venefica* (female) were used interchangeably to denote one who uses poison and to accuse persons of malefic magic. In the pagan world, magic was a common practice; however, using magic against important individuals went against the will of the gods. It was considered a serious crime, and laws were written forbidding its use in these instances.

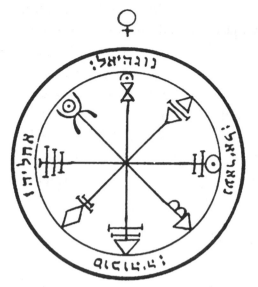

First pentacle of Venus from the Key of Solomon. It is used for obtaining grace and honor, for all things that belong to Venus, and for accomplishing one's desires.

The knowledge of plants and their use in magic and medicine was the domain of the goddess Venus, a goddess connected to the beauty of nature. This included knowledge of poisonous plants as well. Like the goddess herself, nature holds the power to give life and also to take it away. This dual concept of creation and destruction can be seen in the two aspects of goddesses connected to the Venusian current. On the one hand, they are beautiful and nurturing, representing the generative powers of Earth, giving life to both humans and animals. On the other hand, they are the goddesses of destruction, of battle and death. Venus is there at the beginning of life and the end. It is the darkness of the Great Goddess, the primordial chaos of potential, that all life springs from and inevitably returns to. This cycle of birth, life, and death is one of the great mysteries of the Great Goddess.

That is the nature of the plants of Venus. Many of them are both poison and panacea. The same plant can ease suffering and relieve both physical and spiritual sickness or cause death or madness when taken in the wrong quantity or the wrong context. The active chemicals of many of these plants have been used in modern medicine and are still used today to create some of our most important medications. Others have fallen into the wrong hands and have created an epidemic of addiction and spiritual sickness. Many of the plants of Venus are well known for their use as aphrodisiacs, and some are visionary plants that induce the shamanic ecstasy sought by mystics looking to catch a glimpse of the universe. Unlike the dark and dangerous Saturnian plants connected to the dead and the shape-shifting plants of Mercury, the plants of Venus connect with us on an emotional level. They bring healing and empowerment through a synthesis of their divine and chthonic natures. Some of the plants ruled by Venus belong to the same genus as their more sinister counterparts but have a marked distinction in their spiritual natures. Both types of plants can bring gnosis to the botanical magician and wanderer of the Poison Path.

HERBS OF VENUS
Mandrake · Foxglove · Datura · Yarrow · Poppy ·
Dittany of Crete · Vervain

Physical Characteristics
The following characteristics are drawn from Culpeper's *The Complete Herbal*.

> **Leaves:** large and handsome, bright, rich green or roseate, soft and plentiful
>
> **Flowers:** pleasing to the eye, white, blue, rosy, charming, fine, and abundant
>
> **Roots:** of early growth but not deeply fixed, quickly and freely produced
>
> **Odor:** subtle, delightful, pungent, and refreshing to the brain

Medicinal Properties
Venusian herbs are soothing, nourishing tonics for body and spirit and are used for beautification. They are healing balms that nourish and balance all organ systems, promoting harmony within the whole. They are typically

neutral, having both cooling and warming properties. Herbs used in cosmetics, promoting the health of the hair and skin, and luxuriant botanicals are ruled by Venus. Venusian herbs are used in self-care. They promote cellular health and reproduction. Herbs that affect the heart, euphoric herbs, aphrodisiacs, and reproductive toners all have Venusian qualities. Women's health herbs in particular are ruled by Venus. They are energetically harmonizing, helping to center us and open our hearts. Venus helps us attract what we desire and lends her energy to manifestation.

Astrological Correspondences

The following correspondences are drawn from *Practical Astrology for Witches and Pagans* (Dominguez 2016, 60, 62).

Taurus: fixed earth

Second house: inherent talents and powers, what comes naturally, relationship to prosperity, worldly goods and physical body, self-care and beauty

Libra: cardinal air

Seventh house: magical partnerships, covens, how we embody the divine, mediumship and channeling, personal nemesis, how we relate to tutelary spirits

Alchemical Symbolism: Albedo

The second stage is the stage of whiteness, a stage of purification when all blackness disappears and white emerges from the darkness, when the putrefied matter is reduced to ash and calcined to the point that it turns white. Matter attains a fixedness that fire can no longer destroy. It is in this stage that the male and female are united, and the child is born. Albedo is a stage of self-clarity and pure awareness. This stage is ruled by Venus and the moon, represented by the white eagle, dove, or swan. The intermediate stage between nigredo and albedo is also ruled by Venus. It is called the "peacock's tail" for the explosion of colors that occur before the transition. This stage brings us liberation from the shadow, which has become fully integrated.

In alchemy, Venus represents the albedo stage of transmutation, the white phase of calcination, the discovery of the hermaphroditic nature of man. Albedo emerges deep inside the nigredo phase of blackening, represented by the sun rising at midnight. It is the brightest light found within the deepest darkness. It is also Venus in its Morning Star aspect, rising in the dark morning sky, bringing with her the light of the sun.

⚜

Mandrake (*Mandragora officinarum*): Apple of Venus

The mandrake or mandragora is quite possibly the most well-known magical plant in the Western Hemisphere, and maybe even the world. It has made its way into the collective consciousness as a symbol of magic and enchantment, appearing in fairy tales and popular culture. The mandrake and its powers have been known to humankind for thousands of years. It has gone by many names and was present in many cultures, originating in Mesopotamia. The lore of the mandrake preceded its arrival in Europe, where it was first cultivated in 1562 by the herbalist William Turner. The

Mandragora officinarum glyph

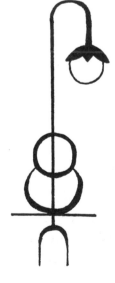

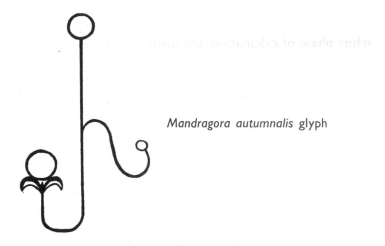

Mandragora autumnalis glyph

alraune, or manikins, of Germanic witches existed throughout Europe prior to the introduction of mandrake. It's likely they created their manikins from white bryony roots. Eventually, their lore was combined with the imported stories of the mandrake.

Over the centuries there has been some confusion between mandrake and its relatives. The categories of mandrake and its taxonomic circumscriptions have also changed. It was known by the name *Atropa mandragora* when the herbalist Carl Linnaeus decided to include it in the *Atropa* genus in his *Species Plantarum,* but there are now two main varieties: *Mandragora officinarum* and *Mandragora autumnalis.*

Mandragora officinarum flowers are greenish white and grow to about one inch in length, in contrast to the violet flowers of *Mandragora autumnalis,* which grow slightly larger. The berries of *M. officinarum* are more globose, and those of *M. autumnalis* are ellipsoid. The seeds of *M. officinarum* are half the size of those of *M. autumnalis,* each berry of the latter containing only a few seeds.

In the 1820s, Antonio Bertoloni distinguished between the spring-blooming *M. vernalis* and the autumn-blooming *M. autumnalis.* His predecessor Dioscorides saw them as male and female mandrakes. Since the 1990s, three circumscriptions have been used to describe this variable perennial. Circumscription is the content of a taxon, a group of one or more organisms that are related and form a unit, such as a species or genus.

The first circumscription identified spring-flowering mandrake as *M. officinarum*, a rarer species confined to northern Italy and the coast of the former Yugoslavia (Jackson and Berry 1979), while *M. autumnalis* referred to most other Mediterranean mandrakes. In 1998, a statistical analysis of morphological characteristics concluded that *M. officinarum* was a single variable species that included *M. autumnalis* (Ungricht et al. 1998). A molecular phylogenic study in 2010 separated the two, regarding *M. officinarum* as the main species, while plants native to the Levant were *M. autumnalis* (Tu et al. 2010). There is no difference in alkaloid content between the two varieties (Thomas and Wentzel 1898).

The name *mandrake* is likely derived from Middle English, alluding to its manlike shape and magical associations. The "man-dragon" was known to the ancient Greeks by the name *circeium* and was associated with Hecate and the sorceress Circe. Superstitions surrounding the mandrake originate with the ancient Greeks, who were aware of the poisonous nature of the mandrake and its relatives. It is part of the nightshade family, the Solanaceae, a group of plants whose members all have their own reputation as magical plants.

The earliest mentions of a plant resembling the mandrake appear in the Book of Genesis and the Song of Solomon. It was used by the Jewish people as a cure for childlessness. The plant was said to glow at night with an otherworldly light known in Hebrew as *baras,* "the fire or the burning." It is referred to as *duda'im* in Genesis 30:14, a word that in the kabbalah relates to soul and spirit or two things united in love and friendship. This is an interesting correlation given the use of the root as a familiar spirit.

Ibn Beithor, an Arab herbalist, refers to mandrake as "the devil's candle," referring to its nocturnal luminosity, which may be explained by the presence of glow worms eating the leaves. In Arabic it was known as devil's lamp and *bayd al-jinn,* meaning "djinn's eggs" or "testes of demons," because of the globose shape of its fruit.

In Rome, mandrake was called *mala terrestria,* meaning "earth's apple." Some of the earliest accounts of mandrake's use in medicine were recorded by the ancient Greeks. The plant was already familiar to the ancients when Hippocrates asserted that "a small dose in wine, less than would occasion delirium, will relieve the deepest depression and anxiety," as mentioned by C. J. S. Thompson in *The Mystic Mandrake*. Interestingly, Aphrodite was referred to as Mandragoritis by the Greeks, meaning "she of the Mandrake."

One of the most well-known traits of the mandrake in folklore is its scream; in Russian, it is called *pevenka trava,* meaning "the plant that screams." This characteristic may have been used as a deterrent, a reference to its powerful nature, or the difficulty in exhuming its large root. Nonetheless, many rituals pertaining to the successful harvest of the mandrake root developed over time. Theophrastus was the one to write the first description of the arcane rites used in harvesting the mandrake, intended to avoid being bewitched by the plant. He wrote his first treatise on plants around 230 BCE. The rituals he described have provided the structure around which many other magical proscriptions have evolved. Some of the practices Theophrastus describes are tracing three circles around the plant with a sword, cutting off the aerial parts of the plant while facing west, and performing ritual and dancing around the site before harvesting the root. It was also deemed necessary to anoint one's hands and face with oil prior to harvesting the root, perhaps as a protective barrier against the plant's juices. Standing upwind would also protect the harvester from noxious spirits since contagion was believed to travel through the air.

As an herb of Venus, mandrake could only be harvested on Friday, the day identified with the goddess, and harvesters adhered to many of the aforementioned ritual superstitions. The root was dug up before sunrise because this was the time when the plant was most active in producing its magical principles and the evil spirit guarding it was asleep. Once collected, the mandrake would be placed in a running stream for a full day and night to remove its diabolical influences. It was then kept wrapped in white cloth in a wooden box.

Dioscorides, the father of pharmacology, investigated hundreds of herbs, including the mandrake. In an illustration in one of his manu-scripts, Heuresis, the goddess of discovery, is depicted giving him the mandrake. It was Dioscorides who suggested the term *mandragora* be adopted for the plant and described its male and female forms.

The mandrake is a prime example of an herb of bewitchment; in every culture where it has left its mark, the plant has been given arcane associations. It is known to be possessed by a spirit, like all plants; how-ever, the spirit of the mandrake is willing to act as a familiar spirit to those who know its rituals. As a plant of Venus, it has been used as an aphrodisiac, an ingredient in love charms and potions, and also as an aid in bestowing fertility. The most important and prized part of the mandrake, the root, gathers its power while it lives in the earth, and so it has a direct connection to the underworld. The root falls under the domain of Saturn, and the plant has been associated with witches, the devil, and a legion of malefic spirits.

Hildegard von Bingen was the first to denounce the mandrake in her writing, describing it in *Physica* as "warm and somewhat watery and is spread by the ground from which Adam was created, it somewhat resembles a person. Because of its similarity to a person there is more diabolical whispering than with other plants and it lays snares for him. For this reason, a person is driven by his desires, whether they are good or bad, as he once did with the idols . . . it is harmful through much that is corruptive of the magicians and phantoms, as many bad things were caused by the idols" (Hildegard 1998, 1.56).

The plant was known to the ancients for its powerful anodyne (pain-relieving) and soporific (sleep-inducing) capabilities. It was often added to wine and paired with opium to be taken as an anesthetizing inebriant. It was known as the soporific sponge or *spongia somnifera,* which was used in the ancient world as an early form of anesthetic. Mandrake and other solanaceous plants were used in medicine up until the 1800s, and in some instances, their active components are still used in pharmaceutical medication.

Mandrake is most famous in magical lore for its use as a manikin or fetish. The prized root in its humanoid form was often carved to

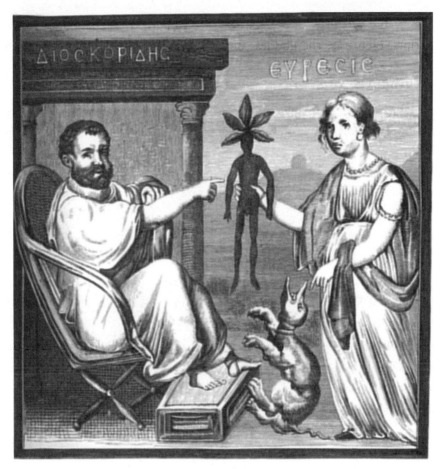

Image of Dioscorides receiving the mandrake from
Heuresis, the goddess of discovery

(From Middleton, *Illuminated Manuscripts in Classical and Mediaeval Times*,
after the Anicia Juliana Codex of Dioscorides in Venice)

increase its resemblance to a man or woman. The root was kept and
treated with reverence, wrapped in fabric and fed with offerings of
wine, milk, honey, and blood. Paul Huson, in *Mastering Witchcraft,*
details the rituals of harvesting the mandrake and its preparation.

The root acts as a vessel for the spirit inhabiting it and has been
known to serve the bearer as a familiar. It can teach one the secrets of
the spirit world, specifically techniques for working with other plants.
They act as intermediaries between the witch and other potential

spiritual allies and can be sent to carry out spells over long distances. Like other poisonous plants, the mandrake is connected to death and the spirit world. It was thought to spring up out of the final void of fluids from those hung at the gallows.

In the fifteenth and sixteenth centuries, the plant was called *Galgemannlein* in Germany, meaning "little man of the gallows." Germanic instructions for caring for the little gallows man, according to C. J. S. Thompson, were as follows: "Wash him clean in red wine, and then wrap him in layers of white and red silk. Lay him in a casket and do not forget firstly to bathe him every Friday, and secondly and more importantly at the new moon to clothe him in a new white shirt" (Thompson 1968, 165).

Mandragora is a patron plant of witches and a powerful ally in their craft. According to Apuleius, the Thessalian witches knew how to bring the mannakin to life so that it could go out and wreak havoc. Although difficult to grow, this plant will thrive for those who are diligent about tending to it. When the time comes and the appropriate rituals and sacrifices are carried out, the spirit of the plant matures and will serve as a protector and teacher for years to come. Mandrake roots have often been passed down through generations, kept in the family for the blessings of prosperity and power that they bring to their stewards.

Roots in general are powerful magical objects that contain the quintessence of the plant. Other roots are also capable of making strong fetishes and take to being carved into humanoid shapes for the creation of homunculi. White bryony has been used throughout northern Europe for similar purposes as the mandrake. This plant, which is more common throughout northern Europe, was sold as a substitute for the rarer mandragora by merchants seeking to benefit from the popularity of the root. Master root, angelica root, poke root, and orris root are a few other examples of plants with large taproots that have been frequently employed for their magical properties. The common dandelion also has a strong earthy root with connections to the lower realms and divination; it is a plant with both a solar and a lunar nature.

Mandrake Dosages and Preparation

While mandrake is a potent entheogen with thousands of years of ritual and lore backing it up, it is one of the safer nightshades to work with. Due to its prominent place in herbal lore and its long history with humanity, mandrake, if acquired, is more willing to work with humans as an ally than its more capricious sisters, belladonna and datura (thorn apple).

However, the plant contains potent tropane alkaloids, and the usual precautions should be taken. Like other members of the nightshade family, mandrake has atropine, scopolamine, apoatropine, l-hyoscyamine, mandragorine, cuscohygrine, norhyoscyamine (soladrine), and belladonnine (in the dried root). Prior to modern chemical analysis, this mixture of alkaloids was referred to collectively as mandragorine. Scopolamine is the primary active component. The root itself contains the majority of the plant's alkaloids. The dried root contains between 0.2 and 0.6 percent alkaloids (Rätsch 2005, 355). The tropane alkaloids present in the fresh root are 0.3 to 0.4 percent by weight. The leaves and fruit contain lower amounts of alkaloids. It was once believed that the fruits were poisonous, but they actually contain only a tiny amount of alkaloids.

Mandrake is grown in the Levant, where the fresh fruits are eaten and used in cooking, and these fruits have been eaten with no overdoses reported. Mandrake, like henbane, is also used in making beer and wine and thus can be safely ingested in this way. The alkaloids in mandrake are soluble in alcohol and water and can be infused in wine or made into a tea. It is suggested when brewing a tea to start with one gram of root and increase from there. Mandrake leaf can be used in smoking blends, and the root can be burned as incense with very subtle effects to both.

Typically, it is only the root that is used in entheogenic preparations, while the aerial parts may be reserved for incense, ritual anointing oils, and other magical applications. The root can be made into a tincture, infused in an oil or ointment, or burned as an incense. Mandrake is the only nightshade, except for henbane, that can be applied to mucous membranes in the form of an oil or ointment; however, these areas more readily absorb ointments and so caution is advised.

Mandrake's effects are hypnotic and intoxicating. In larger doses, it becomes more hallucinogenic. The root burned as an incense creates mild psychoactive effects, while thirty to fifty drops of mother tincture is a psychedelic aphrodisiac (Roth 2017). Medicinal doses of mandrake tincture start at ten drops taken in a glass of water.

Mandrake Plant Spirit Glyphs

Some plants are difficult to come by if they do not grow natively in your area. Mandrake is a perfect example of this; unless you live in the Mediterranean or Middle East you are unlikely to stumble across any. In this case, the glyph (see pages 110–11) can be a wonderful way to connect with the plant.

Foxglove (*Digitalis purpurea*): The Fairy Realm

Foxglove, or *Digitalis purpurea,* one variety of the plant, has gone by many names that indicate its connection with the fairy realm and the beings that populate it. It was called finger flower and, in German, finger-hut for its thimble-like shape. It was also known as goblin's gloves, fairy gloves or caps, witch's thimble, and witches' bells. In Ireland, the tall plant was known as *lusmore,* meaning "the great herb." It originally belonged to the Scrophulariaceae family, known as the figworts, which have similar characteristics, including square stems, opposing leaves, and two-petaled flowers. It now belongs to the large family Plantaginaceae.

According to *Plant Lore, Legends and Lyrics,* the genus name *Digitalis,* from the Latin *digitale,* meaning "thimble or finger stall," was given to the plant in 1542. It was also referenced to a medieval instrument known as the *tintinnabulum,* constructed of a ring of bells hanging on an arched support, which the plant resembles.

It was said that fairies hid inside the large cuplike flowers of the

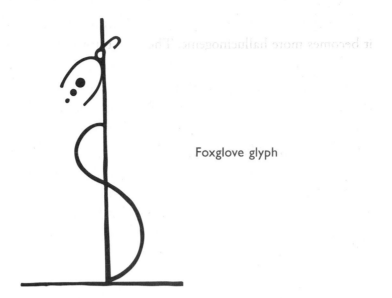

Foxglove glyph

foxglove, and a bent stalk denoted the presence of supernatural beings, weighing down the plant. Foxglove is a biennial woodland plant that produces flowers in its second year. The recognizable purple-pink bells are often seen in works of art depicting fairies and other magical creatures, often alongside the magic mushroom *Amanita muscaria*. Foxglove, like the magic mushroom, is connected to the otherworld by its visionary properties and assists one in communicating with beings from this realm.

The plant is Venusian in nature, denoted by its lush leaves and bell-shaped flowers but more so through its action on the heart. As a homeopathic remedy, it is used for healing the heart and emotional body, bringing love into the aura. It helps dispel fear by bringing strength and courage. It is also used to bring a sense of comfort to those who feel unloved and abandoned. Chemically, the plant produces a poison called digitoxin, which has a powerful effect on the heart, causing a dramatic cardiac response. It is still used in modern medicine in certain heart medications, although rarely. It has been used to treat congestive heart failure and arrhythmias. Even in small doses, the toxins of this plant can cause cardiac arrest and heart failure.

In this sense, Saturn is not the only ruler of botanical poisons. Venus is connected to *veneficia,* for which the crime of poisoning was named, including aphrodisiacs and abortifacients, in addition to being synonymous with witchcraft and sorcery.

In magical practice, this otherworldly herb can be employed in matters of love. The fresh flowers may be used in spells that open one's heart to the idea of love, while dried flowers may be used for the opposite. The extracted juice can be used to charm objects for protection against malicious fairies and other spirits. It can also be used in charms for astral flight and journeying to the underworld where the king and queen of Elphame rule. The queen of Elphame, the fairy queen, is an important figure in traditional witchcraft. She and her consort, the king, rule over the people of Goda, as they are known in the initiatory tradition based on the teachings of Robert Cochrane, the Clan of Tubal Cain. Charms of foxglove protect the bearer, allowing him or her to pass into this realm and return safely. Alternatively, the juice from the plant can be used to negate the harshness of iron blades when their use is desired in conjunction with the more delicate powers of nature.

The cuplike flowers can be used fresh to hold small amounts of milk and honey meant as offerings for the fair folk. Ensorcelled water held within this natural container may be used to anoint the eyelids to better peer into their world. Another sacrament, known as the Rite of the Poisoned Chalice, may be enacted with the aid of foxglove flowers as sacred vessels. In this ritual, a small amount of water is drunk from this tiny floral cup to ritually imbibe the energy of the plant. The bell-shaped flowers may also be strung along a thread and hung as an offering when working spells of glamour and enchantment, for which the fair folk are most adept.

In the eighteenth century, women of the lower classes found an inexpensive, and dangerous, intoxicant in foxglove, drinking tea brewed from this plant. In addition to the potent cardiotoxins, the plant contains highly active glycosides, which are extremely dangerous when isolated. In plant form, the compounds are less potent than when isolated, but they are still dangerous poisons. Ornamental strains of *D. purpurea* contain lower quantities of the active compounds. Foxglove is a counter-toxin to wolfsbane and can be considered just as potent.

Low doses of digitalin, one of the glycosides found in foxglove, are still used today in medicinal preparations. However, the medicinal dose and the toxic dose are precariously close. Just 0.3 g of dried leaves can be toxic to adults. Symptoms of poisoning include dizziness, vomiting, cardiac arrythmia, delirium, hallucinations, and seeing blue. Foxglove is a beautiful plant to grow, and it is a potent magical herb with many applications, but ingesting foxglove in any way should be avoided.

Datura (*Datura stramonium*): The Devil's Weed

The folk names for *Datura stramonium,* and other varieties of this member of the nightshade family, such as *D. inoxia* and *D. metel,* are many: thorn apple, jimson weed, devil's weed, devil's trumpet, devil's breath, raving nightshade, stinkweed, hell's bells, green dragon, and hippomanes. The last was coined by Theocritus for the madness it caused in horses when they ingested the plant. There are eleven currently accepted varieties of *Datura.** Its close relative *Brugmansia* also comes in many different species. They all have experienced some kind of ceremonial use, with *Brugmansia* species being included in ayahuasca ceremonies.

References to this plant in folklore, medieval superstition, and the practice of sorcery are many, and it has made its mark on nearly every continent. This plant is known to many indigenous cultures for its sacred properties and is used as a visionary herb for shamanic rituals by shamans in North and South America. Datura is often associated with the coyote spirit, thought to represent the first shaman. Most shamanic uses of datura across the Americas are magically oriented. It is used in diagnosing, healing, and soul retrieval and is sometimes combined with

---

*Datura, capitalized and italicized, refers to the genus. The same word lowercased and in roman (datura) is a common name used for these plants, primarily *D. stramonium.*

other herbs such as tobacco and fly agaric. Visions induced by datura are particularly important and often lead the initiate to find their spirit animal. It is an important ritual entheogen to many indigenous cultures across the Americas. It has also been used by these cultures in weather magic to appease the spirits to bring rain.

The origins of datura are difficult to determine, though it is seemingly native to North America. Some sources say that it was brought to Europe by the gypsies (Roma) when they migrated there from eastern Europe. "The seeds [of datura] are used as fumigants to chase away ghosts or invoke spirits. All of the gypsies' arts are said to come primarily from a precise knowledge of the juices of the Thorn Apple" (Perger 1864, cited in Rätsch 2005, 209), while other sources say that it was indigenous to the eastern part of North America and brought back to Europe by the early explorers. Either way, this plant has held a major role in the herbal lore of every culture that has cultivated it.

It was used in ancient Greece by the priests of Apollo to enter prophetic states (Schultes, Hofmann, and Rätsch 1992).

Datura has been weaponized, its madness-inducing properties used in ancient chemical warfare. Datura with its tropane alkaloids has been put to many nefarious uses and is known as devil's breath by those who fear it. Jimson weed once incapacitated an entire army that unwittingly ate the plant, leaving the troops out of their minds for days. It was a well-known witching herb in medieval Europe and has been used by prostitutes and thieves for the amnesiac effects it had on their victims.

In India, datura is used in a religious setting to decorate the shrines of deities, but it also has a sinister side and has been used extensively in criminal activity. The madman, the deceiver, and the fool are all associated with the effects of datura. In India, worshippers of the goddess Kali known as *thugs* were thought to have used datura not only in criminal activity but also to drug sacrificial victims.

It continues to be used in the modern era to commit crimes. Its hypnotic, amnesiac, and euphoric effects make victims complacent, prone to suggestion, and incapable of thinking for themselves. It acts as a kind of truth serum, allowing for information to be extracted from its victims, and is also one of the ingredients in Haitian zombie formulas. Haitian zombie powders are surrounded with trepidation and are used only by the *bokor*—a sorcerer. These formulas make use of a specially tailored combination of neurotoxins that keep the victim in a dissociative state. After initially drugging the victim and putting him into a deathlike sleep, the bokor would often bury the victim. After disinterring the traumatized victim a couple of days later, the bokor would continue drugging the victim to keep him in a subservient state.

Datura is a plant of the nocturnal garden, along with other plants associated with the moon, sleep, and the psychic realm. It can be used to honor the primeval goddess Nyx, who is an embodiment of the night, and her children, Hypnos, Morpheus, and Thanatos, the gods of sleep, dreams, and death. Datura rules the night and is associated with nocturnal creatures, such as the moth, owl, and wolf.

Datura blossoms point upward toward the night sky, like trumpets from the underworld, the nocturnal flowers opening at dusk. The blossoms are sometimes called moonflowers and resemble the night-blooming moon vine *Ipomoea alba,* a tropical morning glory. In the evening hours, datura sends out from its flowers a sweet and intoxicating aroma, which is said to be capable of inducing trance. Datura's relative *Brugmansia* is called angel's trumpet because its flowers point downward from the heavens. As part of the nocturnal realm, thorn apple is a dreaming plant, used to gain the power of divination and soul flight. The flowers can be placed around the bed of a person who is trying to dream prophetically. As a psychic herb of lunar nature, it awakens the crown and third eye, enhancing psychic ability and clarity and giving insight into the meaning of dreams. It can also be used to ward off nightmares and for protection during sleep.

Like the other baneful herbs in the nightshade family, datura is strongly connected with death, the underworld, nocturnal forces, dark practices, and the dark goddess. As a visionary plant, it opens the gateways to both the upper and lower realms for us to travel. It helps us

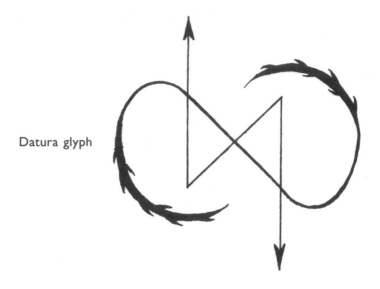

Datura glyph

process fear and anxiety surrounding death and can be burned to banish malevolent spirits and for breaking hexes, specifically those that plague the victim in his or her sleep. It is a powerful ally in soul retrieval and the reversal of ancestral curses. It is used homeopathically against restlessness, terror, and delusions.

Its connections to Venus are via the tropane alkaloids, which can cause intense arousal, euphoria, and suggestibility. It can also be used in formulas of manipulation and coercion in love spells of a more controlling nature. Like their relatives in the Solanaceae family, the various species of datura contain tropane alkaloids, typically atropine, hyoscyamine, daturine, stramonine, and scopolamine. Scopolamine, which causes memory loss, is responsible for the amnesiac effects that this plant is known for. It is used in modern medicine to treat motion sickness and during surgery. Datura has a decreased alkaloid content during the day and a higher content at nighttime (Lewin 1998). This is an interesting physical manifestation of datura's connection to the night. It can cause death by respiratory failure and heart attack. As a user builds up tolerance in the nervous system to datura's hallucinogenic effects, larger doses are required to achieve the same effect, but these higher doses have an increasingly deleterious effect on the heart. When used too frequently, the tropane alkaloids can build up in the cardiac tissues, causing an overdose.

Scopolamine poisoning causes low brain waves but prevents deep sleep. This places one in a waking dreamlike state. Early experiments conducted by Andrés Laguna with the help of Giambattista della Porta were performed using salves to show that supernatural journeys were just dreams. He notes how men drank potions of datura to create the illusion of being a bird or a beast and that they donned wolfskins while running around on all fours (Siegel 1989).

While datura is a powerful and seductive ally in the craft of the poisoner, it can quickly turn on its user, causing madness, coma, and death. The utmost caution should be taken when working with this powerful plant spirit and its alkaloids. Extensive research and controlled experimentation are key in making informed decisions about the ritual use of this plant and its relatives.

Datura Dosages and Preparation

Medicinally, datura has many uses, from the treatment of rheumatism and pain to hair loss, abortion, healing wounds, inflammation, nervous disorders, and opium overdose. Medicinal usage of *Datura* varieties was common in many cultures. It was believed that when taken medicinally it would not result in supernatural powers. Small amounts were taken to treat many illnesses and as aphrodisiacs. It was only through the preparation of the plant with the intent to communicate with spirits paired with ritual that magical access was made available.

In *Pharmako Gnosis,* an important text to followers of the Poison Path, the author, Dale Pendell, notes that datura is grouped in the category called *Daimonica.* He states that while datura may be the single most dangerous visionary plant in North America, it is an interdimensional ally. It allows the visionary to transcend the rules of time and space and commune with the spirit world. Pendell describes the action of the stramonium alkaloids, saying that, at low doses, scopolamine causes cardiac slowing, acting as a sedative; however, at higher doses, it is excitatory to the central nervous system, resulting in hallucinations and restlessness.

The plant material when taken for its entheogenic properties is typically smoked but can also be ingested as a tea or made into an ointment. Richard Miller, in *The Encyclopedia of Magical Herbalism,* suggests that the dried leaves be rolled into cigarettes. The suggested dosage is two cigarettes of one gram of plant material each, smoked over a period while monitoring the effects until the desired level of intoxication is achieved. The seeds are said to be most consistent in their alkaloid content, while the rest of the plant varies in toxicity, the highest levels being found in the roots. Symptoms of toxicity occur thirty to sixty minutes after smoking the leaves or drinking tea and one to four hours after ingestion of plant material or seeds. The seeds are the most active chemically at 0.66 percent, maintaining their alkaloid content when dried or boiled. The flowers also have a high alkaloid content, up to 0.61 percent.

Pendell agrees that smoking the leaves is the safest means of ingesting this plant for these purposes, compared to other methods of ingestion. When using the seeds, no more than fifteen would be considered a safe dose. Other sources mention using fewer seeds when making a tea: five to seven seeds crushed and steeped for an hour, with the tea taken thirty minutes prior to ritual. Although this gives us some perspective regarding dosage, it is important to remember the differences in each individual's chemistry and the varying alkaloid content of one plant to another. The alkalinity of these plants is influenced by factors such as the amount of sunlight and nitrogen levels in the soil, which can raise the toxicity of a plant significantly.

The concentration of specific alkaloids is highly variable and depends on environmental factors, growing season, soil, and how the plant material is stored. Toxicity may vary even in a single plant, from one leaf to the next. The highest concentration of alkaloids occurs in the seeds, with approximately 0.1 mg of atropine per seed or 3 to 6 mg atropine per fifty to one hundred seeds (Goldfrank 1994, cited in Arnett 1995). Each seed contains approximately 0.05 mg of scopolamine. As few as seven seeds have resulted in poisoning when ingested. The seedpods are divided into four lobed chambers, each containing fifty to one hundred seeds. A lethal dose of atropine in adults is reached anywhere beyond 10 mg, and the threshold for scopolamine is lower, being greater than 2 to 4 mg (Goodman, cited in Arnett 1995).

Here are various recommended doses for therapeutic and entheogenic purposes from Voogelbreinder (2009).

1 gram smoked as a therapeutic dose for asthma
40 seeds burned on charcoal disks and inhaled for visions
6 flowers added to coffee for a stimulating inebriant

The following recommended medicinal dosages are from Grieve (1971).

0.1–5 grains powdered leaves (equivalent to 6.5–324 mg)
1–3 drops fluid extract from leaves
1–2 drops fluid extract from seeds
5–15 drops tincture of leaves

✿❧

Datura Pain Relief Salve

*This salve can be applied to bumps and bruises
and used to relieve strained and sore muscles.*

- 3 Tbsp. datura seeds
- ½ oz. arnica flowers
- ½ oz. comfrey root
- 1 cup carrier oil
- ¼ cup beeswax or carnauba wax

Make sure all of the ingredients you are using are dry before infusing them in oil. Cook the datura seeds, arnica flowers, and comfrey root in the oil over medium heat in a slow cooker or double boiler for 4 hours. Strain out the plant material before adding the beeswax. Once you add the beeswax you may have to turn up the heat or switch to the stovetop to melt the wax.

⚜

Thorn Apple Tincture (Church and Church 2009)

- ⚘ 1 part *Datura stramonium* leaves and flowering tops
- ⚘ 10 parts 45 percent alcohol

Harvest the leaves and flowering tops in July. Macerate the plant material in the alcohol for two to three weeks. Dosage is 5–10 ml per week.

⚜

Yarrow (*Achillea millefolium*): Ancient Herb of Love and War

This common plant, known as thousand leaf, arrowroot, woundwort, bloodwort, and staunch grass, is a powerful ally in an unassuming package. Yarrow has been used for its blood-clotting and protective properties for centuries. It has been found in Neanderthal burial sites in Iraq dating back to 60,000 BCE. It is named *Achillea millefolium* for the ancient warrior who is credited with its creation. It is said that Achilles created the plant from the iron rust scraped from his spear, which he used to heal one of his soldiers. Since then, yarrow has been a patron of warriors, a protector during battle and giver of courage. Medicinally, it assists in the clotting of blood and is used in poultices to stop bleeding and to assist the healing of wounds. It is antiseptic, astringent, anti-inflammatory, and analgesic, making it an all-purpose herb of healing. Not only is it a panacea for humans, but it also benefits surrounding plants through its root secretions, which strengthen and protect its neighbors.

Yarrow contains several interesting compounds, including thujone, the chemical found in wormwood that is used to make absinthe, which is also found in mugwort, juniper, and common sage. It also contains glycoalkaloids, which are present in bittersweet nightshade and potato plants, as well as achilleine, another type of alkaloid. Although alkaloids are present, the plant is not considered poisonous. The essential oil has a bluish color like that of chamomile, which is attributed to the presence of azulene, which turns blue when distilled.

Its spiritual and ritual uses are just as indispensable as its healing capabilities. It is an herb associated with both Venus and Mars and elemental water and fire. It strengthens the aura and establishes boundaries by creating balance between opposing forces. It is a plant of both the healer and the warrior, used to heal energetic and physical wounds, sealing holes in the aura and adjusting its size and permeability. It is perfect for those who are exposed to foreign energies via spiritual work and healing. Allowing the aura to expand or contract, it enhances its ability to block or facilitate energy flow. It can be used in tandem with labradorite, a stone with similar properties, to protect against astral parasites, energy vampires, and attachments.

Yarrow is all about boundaries and helps us determine if something isn't good for us, giving us a sense of protection and reducing anxiety. It is also beneficial when establishing healthy boundaries with other people. The plant is especially useful for those who are empathetic and whose energies are easily influenced and depleted by others. Yarrow also enhances our own ability to heal while protecting us from environmental influences.

As one of the nine sacred herbs of Midsummer's Eve, Yarrow has many magical uses as well. Not only does it act as a powerful ward, keeping unwanted things at bay, it also allows for what is desirable to pass through uninhibited. Yarrow sticks are known for their use in the divinatory practice of the I Ching. It aids in psychic awareness by enhancing energy flow and blocking out unwanted chatter, allowing messages to come through more clearly. It is a magical catalyst that potentiates other herbs and has been used in spells to break curses and impart courage and in exorcism. Yarrow has been widely used as an ingredient in love spells and for drawing the attention of someone one wishes to see.

Thousand leaf seems to have a thousand uses and is proof that the simplest of plants are often the most ancient and useful herbal allies. It has helped humankind for centuries. Today, such herbs are considered weeds by those who do not know the many secrets that they hold.

Poppy (*Papaver somniferum*): The Gateway of Life and Death

HYPNOS: THE FUMIGATION FROM A POPPY

Sleep, king of Gods, and men of mortal birth,
Sov'reign of all sustain'd by mother Earth;
For thy dominion is supreme alone,
O'er all extended, and by all things known.
'Tis thine all bodies with benignant mind
In other bands than those of brass to bind:
Tamer of cares, to weary toil repose,
From whom sweet solace in affliction flows.
Thy pleasing, gentle chains preserve the soul,
And e'en the dreadful cares of death controul;
For Death and Lethe with oblivious stream,
Mankind thy genuine brothers justly deem.
With fav'ring aspect to my pray'r incline,
And save thy Mystics in their works divine.

ORPHIC HYMN TO HYPNOS (SLEEP), NO. 85

The poppy, *Papaver somniferum*, has been both balm and bane to humankind. Other varieties include *P. album*, *P. nigrum*, and *P. glabra*. It has eased the pain of centuries of humanity's woes, bringing peaceful sleep to the weary. It has also started wars and has become part of an epidemic of individuals looking to escape the pains and worries of human life. The poppy and its opium contain the alkaloids morphine, codeine, and narcotine, which have been synthesized and used to create some of the strongest pain-killing medications of modern medicine. Like heroin, these substances are dangerous and powerfully addictive. They have been created by the pharmaceutical industry for profit without any regard for public safety. The addictive chemicals of the poppy can quickly ensnare its victims, creating a euphoria and numbing the emotions, after which normal functioning quickly becomes unbearable.

Methods for obtaining opium were first discovered in Stone Age central Europe. Remnants have been excavated from Neolithic tombs in France, Switzerland, northern Italy, and southern Germany. Roman accounts claimed that Celtic Gauls were aware of the poppy's cultivation, harvest, and use. In early Germanic lore, poppy fields were known as sacred sites to Odin or Wotan and were visited by pilgrims for healing. It was taken internally to protect against nocturnal creatures, such as vampires, and to ward off nightmares.

Poppy has been part of the world's pharmacopoeia since the most ancient times, when it was propagated in Asia Minor and its use as a medicine spread. Its medicinal value as a powerful pain reliever and sedative has long been known. Paracelsus created the famous remedy laudanum from opium, henbane, crushed pearls, and coral. It was said to be superior to all other remedies. Laudanum was used as a remedy throughout Europe until the late 1600s. The English physician Thomas Sydenham had a similar tincture of opium poppy, saffron, cinnamon, powdered cloves, and Spanish wine. His standardized recipe was an effective remedy for pain and a powerful inebriant known as Sydenham's laudanum.

All varieties of the Papaveraceae family and its relatives contain active alkaloids and have medicinal properties. For example, *P. rhoeas* contains the alkaloid rhoeadine, a mild sedative. Another member of the family is the California poppy, *Eschscholzia californica,* which is native to the United States and Mexico. It acts as a nervous system relaxer, sedative, and pain reliever. Frayed nerves from stress, causing insomnia, can be calmed with a tincture (see dosages and preparation on page 134). It is illegal to collect this flower in the wild in California because it is the state flower, but it is easily grown.

The poppy is a plant of the moon, the underworld, and the place between life, death, and sleep. The milky latex of the poppy was known as "tears of the moon." Theocritus tells us that poppies grew from the spilled tears of Aphrodite as she mourned the death of Adonis. Poppies are associated with the sphere of Binah, which represents the void of creation. They are associated with the mother and crone aspect of the Great Goddess. Both Cybele and Ceres are associated with poppies and are often depicted holding or wearing them. The goddess Nyx had poppies around her temples.

Ancient Greek mythology placed the origins of poppy with the goddess Ceres (Greek) or Demeter (Roman), who is attributed with growing the flower after her daughter Persephone (Kore in the Greek myth) was abducted by Hades. Some myths say that Demeter grew the flower after her daughter was taken so that she might sleep and forget her pains. Other stories say that Persephone was in a field picking poppies at the time of her abduction before becoming the queen of the underworld. As a crop, poppies were grown in succession to wheat and barley, which was also sacred to Ceres-Demeter. The goddess is often depicted holding both plants. Hypnos, Hermes, and Thanatos were also shown holding the flower or pod because of the plant's connection to sleep and death. Morpheus, the son of Nyx,

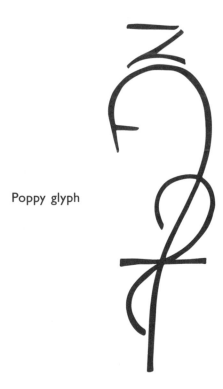

Poppy glyph

was the god of dreams, and it was from him that morphine derived its name.

The poppy is a plant of the realm of the dead and was used by Romans in offerings to appease the spirits of the dead. It was called the Lethean poppy by Virgil in reference to the River Lethe or Ameles Potamos, "river of unmindfulness," one of the five rivers of the underworld. The River Lethe flowed through the underworld around the cave of Hypnos and caused forgetfulness in all who drank its waters. The river is crossed by the newly dead as they descend into the underworld and forget their former lives. The common poppy, *Papaver rhoeas,* was the first plant to come back in the battlefields in northern France and Belgium after World War I. It became the symbol of remembrance for fallen soldiers.

As a plant of the night and the moon, the poppy rules over dreams, illusions, and shadows. The seeds of the plant are used in hexes to cause confusion and forgetfulness. They are also used in workings to blind one's enemies. When used for cursing, the flowers are gathered in the enemy's name. They can alternatively be used to send dreams and visions and to draw down the influence of the moon. Lunacy or madness is associated with the moon and its influence when it is full. The petals of the flowers can also be used in charms for luck in love, money, and health.

Papaver somniferum is often one of the ingredients listed in medieval flying ointments and was likely included to counteract some of the more uncomfortable side effects of the tropane alkaloids. Opium and its derivatives are said to be antidotes for poisoning by these alkaloids. Decoctions of poppies were made from bruised capsules and distilled water, which were used externally to soothe pain. The juice of the poppy was also included in the *spongia somnifera,* an early form of anesthetic used for surgical operations, which also contained ingredients like mandrake and henbane. The pain-relieving properties of the nightshades offer a nonaddictive alternative to modern opioids. They have also been shown to relieve uncomfortable withdrawal symptoms from these medications, allowing people to taper off them more comfortably.

Poppy Dosages and Preparation

The dried leaves were traditionally made into infusions or decoctions and were also smoked. Poppies were often included in recipes for medieval witches' flying ointments. One example includes poppy, mandrake root, henbane, belladonna berries, and opium juice. This would have created a powerful soporific, which would have resulted in a deep dream-filled sleep.

෴

Tincture of California Poppy
(*Eschscholzia californica*)

All parts of the plant can be used for this tincture, including the flowers, leaves, and roots. Chop up the fresh plant material and then use the "folk tincture" method: Fill your jar with the plant material and cover with high-proof grain alcohol until the plant material is submerged beneath half an inch of liquid. Allow the tincture to macerate for a full lunar cycle, shaking it regularly.

The tincture can be taken to calm nerves, ease pain, and combat insomnia. Start with 5–10 drops before increasing to higher dosages.

For insomnia: Take 20–50 drops or ¼–½ tsp., 1 hour before bed
For pain: Take 40–60 drops over the course of an hour; repeat every 4–6 hours as needed
For anxiety: Take 5–10 drops as needed throughout the day

Dittany of Crete
(*Origanum dictamnus*):
The Love Herb

This species of oregano grows only on the mountainous terrain of the island of Crete. Over time, it has developed a reputation for use in love magic, being fed to lovers to increase their passion.

This old European love herb has also been used in Samhain celebrations because of its ability to manifest spirits, induce trance, and promote clairvoyance. It is known for its use as a ritual incense, which emits a thick smoke that serves as a medium for the physical manifestation of spirits. Author Paul Huson and occultist Aleister Crowley both suggest using it for the visible manifestation of spirits, as well as increasing spirit sight and magical power in general. It can also be used as a wash for crystal balls and other divinatory tools.

Dittany is connected to both Venus and the moon. It is linked to the lunar goddess Diana through the name Diktynna. Much of the modern lore surrounding this plant came from the Theosophical Society, which held it sacred to the moon goddess and valued it for its trance-inducing effects. The root was recommended by the oracle of Phthas. Dittany is associated with the goddess Venus by Virgil in *The Aeneid,* Book XII, which tells of Venus using the plant to heal the wounded hero Aeneas: "Not unknown is that herb to wild goats, when winged arrows have lodged in their flanks." This obscure connection to wild goats has led to the herb being used in incense blends to sylvan gods like Pan. When injured, wild goats were seen seeking out this mountain plant for its healing properties. Plutarch said that the women of Crete, noticing this behavior, learned to make use of the plant in childbirth (Folkard 1884, 165).

Vervain
(*Verbena officinalis*):
Herb of Enchantment

The genus *Verbena* has many varieties. Vervain is called by many names: the sorcerer's herb, the herb of enchantment, herba sacra, and herba Veneris. Known to witches and sorcerers for centuries, it is one of the classical plants associated with magic, particularly love magic. As one of the choice herbs for magic, it has seen extensive use as a magical and alchemical aid throughout history.

It is said to have been used by the Druids in their lustral or holy waters for blessings and libations. A fairy herb, it has been used in rites to summon and honor the fae and nature spirits. The Celts called vervain "the tresses of Taliesin," after the famous mythic bard who received his magical powers from the goddess Cerridwen.

This multipurpose herb can seemingly be used in virtually all forms of practical magic. It can confer protection to the summoner when calling upon spirits. It is strewn around the ritual circle or triangle of manifestation. For a similar effect it can be placed upon the altar. Vervain can also be employed as a visionary herb by being made into an infusion to fill scrying vessels or as a wash for divinatory tools. The herb also helps enhance divination by clearing the mind, centering the spirit, and enhancing psychic ability. Vervain contains iridoids, which are precursors to alkaloids.

As herba Veneris, vervain has a history of use as a popular love herb used in amorous spells and charms. When made into a wash, it is used on the hands before performing love spells for added power. This herb has a unique elemental quality sometimes seeming to manifest all four elements at different times. Like Solomon's seal, it can be used as a general elemental offering, and its affinity with the forces of nature can help keep plants healthy. It can also be used for healing the land and helping to empower the spirits of nature, especially in places where they have been neglected.

Historically, this plant has been used in amulets for both protection and prosperity. An herb of evasion, it can aid one in escaping one's enemies and avoiding detection as it brings qualities of shape-shifting and invisibility to the aura. Spells of obscuration and hiding, whether of living things, places, or objects, fall under the shared rule of Saturn and Venus, based in concealment and glamour.

Vervain is a multipurpose magical catalyst and, as such, a

versatile and powerful ally in the arcane workings of the plant magician. While not all catalysts are poisons or hallucinogens, their effects can enhance spell work, ritual mind-set, and perception through aromatherapeutic effects, such as enhancing mental clarity and memory.

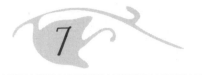

The Book of Mercury
Traversing the Realms

*T*he spirit of Mercury is a teacher and ally to the student of magic, occultism, and esoteric studies, an ever-present spirit taking on many forms. Mercury and the other masks worn by this elder spirit are the patrons of the arcane arts. One notable characteristic of Mercurian spirits is their fluidity. They have the ability to change shape and travel where other beings cannot. They exist outside the confines of space and time. Mercurian spirits are tricksters, shamans, and gatekeepers. They guide us through initiation and transformation, bringing us new perspectives. These figures are often depicted as multifaceted, androgynous, and wild. Among Mercury's many manifestations, as noted in chapter 4, are Prometheus, Loki, Lucifer, and Thoth. The spirits and

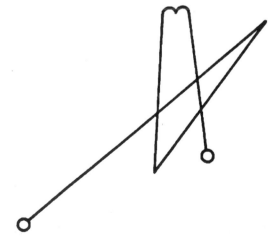

Sigil of the intelligence
of Mercury

(From Agrippa, *Three Books of Occult Philosophy*)

8	58	59	5	4	62	63	1
49	15	14	52	53	11	10	56
41	23	22	44	45	19	18	48
32	34	35	29	28	38	39	25
40	26	27	37	36	30	31	33
17	47	46	20	21	43	42	24
9	55	54	12	13	51	50	16
64	2	3	61	60	6	7	57

Kamea of Mercury
(From Agrippa, *Three Books of Occult Philosophy*)

deities involved often transform from culture to culture, united by similar themes under different names.

Mercury as an elder god, preceding the pantheons and nomenclatures of human civilization, is the wild spirit of nature, having two sides, both dark and light, with many shades of gray in between. He is the spirit of the unknown, the mysterious light in the darkness that when reached fills us with illuminating wisdom, showing us yet another turn on the eternal path. Only by exploring the many masks worn by this primal force do we begin to grasp the true scope of this primal entity. In this chapter, we explore his identity as Thoth, Janus, and the green man, the wild spirit of nature who has connections to the devil.

THOTH: ANCIENT EGYPTIAN GOD OF WRITING, WISDOM, AND MAGIC

The reedy stalk-like stem of *Acorus calamus* was said to have been used by the ancient Egyptian god Thoth to write. Thoth is an earlier counterpart to Hermes and Mercury who shares many similar attributes and sheds light on the origin of this spirit. Thoth, one of the early deities of ancient Egyptian religion, played a major role in the story of creation and the lives of the gods. In Egyptian mythology he is one of the deities who created and maintained the universe. He was later seen as an arbitrator. When disputes between other gods would arise, it was the wisdom and authority of Thoth that would be sought to reach an agreement or find a solution. The fact that the other gods deferred to his ruling is a testament to his important status. In later myth, Thoth was connected to the sacred writing of hieroglyphics, which he was said to have invented. He was also credited with the invention of science and the magical arts. He was perhaps the wisest of all the gods, responsible for the arts and their introduction to humankind.

Thoth as an early incarnation of the messenger archetype was seen as an intermediary spirit in his role of connecting the physical and spiritual realms, and in this role of bringing the knowledge of language, writing, and the sciences to early man. He also played an important role in the judgment of the dead, a role that he shares with his Greco-Roman counterparts who acted as psychopomps leading the dead to the afterlife. Thoth serves as a judge of the dead, weighing their deeds on Earth to determine their fate in the afterlife. The ancient Greeks frequently equated the deities of other cultures with their own gods, when they shared similar characteristics. Such was the case with Hermes and Thoth.

Thoth's symbols are representative of his many various roles, which changed over time. Originally, he was a lunar deity depicted wearing a headdress with a lunar disk when acting in his role as keeper of the calendar. His symbols are the ibis, papyrus, sacred alphabets, writing tools, and scales. The plants used to produce papyrus and the construction of writing utensils came from the wetlands where ibises roamed. His connection with time and cycles is intriguingly Saturnian and related to the role of the previously mentioned Janus. Mercurian spirits often display Saturnian themes in their darker, more chthonic roles.

The most apparent similarities are with Hermes, who oversaw many of the same tasks. The later figure known to alchemists and magicians as Hermes Trismegistus, or Hermes Thrice Great, who is credited with writing numerous magical texts, is a composite of Hermes and Thoth.

Trismegistus was a Greek translation of a title that was originally applied to the god Thoth. Thoth, the thrice great, like later shape-shifting spirits of a mercurial nature, often took many names based on his numerous roles and assumed more than one shape, most often as a man with the head of an ibis or baboon but also in the form of an ibis or ape. The ability of shape-shifting spirits to transform from human to animal or to a combination of both or to have polycephaly (multiple heads) all indicate their boundary-blurring nature.

While Hermes and Mercury are more concerned with travel and communication between the material and spiritual worlds, Thoth rules over communication via sacred writing, specifically hieroglyphics and other magical alphabets. His dominion also extends to the realms of philosophy and religion. He was seen by ancient Egyptians as a cosmic architect. In ancient Egyptian myth, Thoth was self-created and went on to create the first gods and goddesses of the Egyptian pantheon. He used his sacred wisdom and knowledge of the laws of the universe to create the intricate structure that holds the worlds together. It is this connection that we seek to reach through ritual and symbol by selecting specific threads of fate we can manipulate to create change. By representing individual points of creation through symbol and ritual reenactment, we act in the same way as the gods, creating change through will.

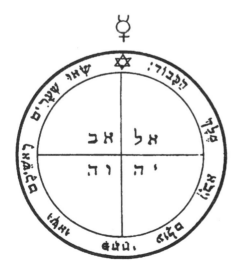

Fifth pentacle of Mercury from the Key of Solomon. It commands the spirits of Mercury and opens all doors, gateways, and fetters, and nothing it encounters may resist it.

MERCURY IN GREEK
AND ROMAN MYTHOLOGY

To the Romans, the ancient god Mercurius was one of the Dii Consentes—twelve major deities of the Roman pantheon that were held in high esteem. Many of these deities predate the Roman Empire and were indigenous to the land. They were referred to as *di indigetes,* a concept also found in ancient Greece describing the most ancient spirits as *autochthonic,* or having always existed as part of the land. Each discovery of an earlier form of these deities leads one to an even more primordial origin of these ancient spirits.

Mercurius became syncretized with the Greek Hermes in the fourth century BCE. In ancient Roman religion, with its Proto-Indo-European roots, we find some of the earliest forms of this spirit, with counterparts in ancient Egypt. In Roman mythology, the spirits known as the Lares were children of Mercurius. These spirits were similar to the modern idea of land spirits, combining the idea of the spirits of a place, or genii loci, with familiar spirits and ancestral spirits. Offerings to these spirits would be made in the home at the hearth or the home's ancestral shrine. Offerings were also made at designated markers, known as *herms.* These sacred places were originally simple stone cairns, piles of stones left as offerings, that would be found at crossroads and boundaries between

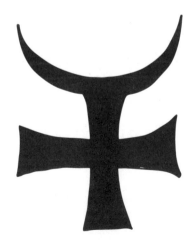

A medieval symbol for Mercury, combining the cross of matter and crescent of spirit. A later addition of the circle, representing the soul, connects the three parts of humanity and the universe.

territories. They were later converted into more permanent structures at these liminal areas where travelers would make offerings in exchange for the spirits' blessing.

Mercury, as messenger of the gods, had the unique ability of being able to travel between all three realms—the upper (celestial), middle (terrestrial), and lower (chthonic). He is an intermediary spirit that rules over crossroads, gateways, and in-between areas. Mercurian spirits are often contacted at the beginning of rituals, being honored first so that they ensure that the working is successful and the message is heard. There is an entire group of beings that fit into the category of gate-keepers, and they hold the keys to traveling to the other worlds. Their ability to change shape and move between realms makes them impor-tant teachers for shamanic workings, astral travel, and acquiring arcane knowledge. In addition to their role as messenger, they rule the arts of communication, language, and the written word. Sacred alphabets and written spells are often attributed to Mercurian spirits, who are often petitioned in such instances. Mercury is a god of alchemy, magic, and all sacred sciences and can assist in these areas.

JANUS, THE TWO-FACED GOD

As with many of the original deities of the religion of ancient Rome, Janus has origins in the pre-Roman religions of the Etruscans, an ancient tribal people who occupied the area before the Roman Empire. Their culture made many of the first contributions to the early beliefs of the Mediterranean. Janus is connected to the Etruscan deity Culsans, who rules over doors and gateways. In Roman mythol-ogy, Janus presides over similar themes, including all thresholds and liminal places, both physical and symbolic. A deity of transitions, rul-ing beginnings and endings, he acts as an initiator. He is depicted with two faces, making him a god of duality, ruling both darkness and light, past and present. He rules over the movements of the sun, stars, and moon. Dianus (Janus) was a god of light, while Diana (Jana) was a goddess of the moon. He is said to rule over the movements of the gods because he is found at all doorways and thresholds where the realms meet. This is the reason that he is invoked first in Roman rituals, before any other god or goddess is petitioned. Similar functions and rituals are ascribed in African diasporic traditions to Elegba, who is also mercurial in nature. Also known as Papa Legba, he is a trickster-type spirit who plays a major role in Vodou religion. Other spirits cannot be contacted without Legba's blessing.

There have been many spirits fulfilling similar functions throughout history that can be connected by their common attributes, namely their dual nature and their tendency to blur the division between these polarities. This concept of dark and light can be found in the most ancient pantheons, including those of Babylon and Sumer. The two-faced gods of antiquity were embodiments of the dark and light halves of the year and the division between night and day, represented by the sun and moon.

Janus was worshipped at planting and harvest times, which were directly connected to the calendar year and the turning of the celestial wheel. The solstices, the points of greatest light and greatest darkness, were some of the most important times around which ancient religions where built.

As noted previously in chapter 4, early myth tells of Saturnus in his original role as an agricultural deity who brought knowledge of planting and harvest to Janus, becoming his friend and ally. After leaving a hostile environment in ancient Greece, Saturn shared rulership of this early Roman kingdom with Janus. It was during the reign of Saturn that the mythical golden age flourished and men lived in harmony with Earth, sharing her bounty. In this original version of Saturn with his scythe, he is a reaper of the fruits of Earth, not the grim reaper harvesting souls. Further research will reveal Janus's connection to the figure of the horned god through an exploration of his Indo-European origins as well as his connection to Saturnus and Mercurius.

THE GREEN MAN:
SPIRIT OF THE WILD

The green man is an ancient concept and dualistic in nature; he represents the creative and destructive aspects of nature. In his Saturnian form, the green man, or green devil, presides over the dark half of the year and the processes of rot and decay so that new life can be born. Alternatively, he is the virile force of procreation, a mischievous and Mercurian spirit depicted as part man, part animal, and part plant. The spirit of the green man is truly a mystery. He represents the sentient force of nature, particularly the verdant spirit of the forest. The green man has been seen in architecture and artwork since the Middle Age, with origins in ancient Rome, Mesopotamia, and Constantinople. He was likely a representation of deities such as Dionysus or Bacchus, Pan, and Sylvanus.

The wild spirit of nature can be found in folklore across Europe in the wild man of the woods known as a *woodwose*. Variations of this spirit can be found in Germany and Switzerland and in the later English figure of Jack in the Green. All these green men are depicted covered in the wild growth of the woodlands, often with vines wrapping around their bodies and coming out of their mouths.

In his darker aspect, the green devil, he represents the "wild adversary" in nature, the spirit of death and decay who resides in the wildwood and rules during the dark half of the year. He is the horned god of the forest who acts as protector and defender of secrets. The green devil can be called upon by those who would seek the occult mysteries of the natural world and ask them to be revealed. As a trickster spirit, he often teaches through riddles and lessons, forcing us to use our own gifts of discernment to make even deeper discoveries. He is a shape-shifter, the virile god of the natural world, the king of beasts and leader of the hunt who also rules the growing half of the year. He then becomes the god of the harvest—sacrificed at the end of the growing season only to be resurrected as the dark god leading the wild retinue of souls through the stormy winter skies.

HERBS OF MERCURY

Fly Agaric · Calamus · Parsley · Lady's Mantle · Greater Periwinkle ·
Wolfsbane · Wild Lettuce · Centaury · Enchanter's Nightshade

Physical Characteristics

The following characteristics are drawn from Culpeper's *The Complete Herbal*.

> **Leaves:** different shapes and kinds that are pleasing to the eye
> **Flowers:** various descriptions and colors that are refreshing, agreeable, and pleasant
> **Roots:** abiding deep in the earth, spreading far and wide
> **Odor:** subtle and penetrating, refreshing to the heart and brain

Medicinal Properties

Mercurian herbs are dualistic in nature, neither masculine nor feminine but a combination, representing both aspects. Mercury rules over the brain, the mind, and the nervous system. It is present in all our mental processes and how we interpret sensory information, our memory, and our language skills. The sensory organs, specifically those involved in communication, are ruled by Mercury. Mercurian herbs are energetic; their effects manifest quickly. They are plants that influence the nervous system and change our mood and our mental processes. These herbs increase mental function whether through stimulation, promoting alertness, or enhancing memory. They are brain herbs or nootropics, substances that improve cognitive function, and are valuable to those whose careers involve writing or speaking. Mercurian herbs also expand our consciousness and allow us to travel between worlds. They help enhance intuition and facilitate meditation. They provide clarity during stressful times in our lives.

Astrological Correspondences

The following correspondences are drawn from *Practical Astrology for Witches and Pagans* (Dominguez 2016, 60, 62).

Gemini: mutable air

Third house: communication, receptivity, telepathy and psychic communication, spoken spells, chanting, incantations, summoning

Virgo: mutable earth

Sixth house: spiritual and magical oaths and contracts, duties, balancing the mundane and spiritual, wyrd and fate, work and health

Alchemical Symbolism: Rubedo

The stage of reddening is the final stage and culmination of the Great Work. It is related to Mercury. It is the chemical wedding and union of male and female, the volatile and fixed aspects of matter and spirit. This is the triumph of the work, the hermaphroditic offspring or philosophical mercury. The philosopher's stone is vital to the completion of the Great Work and is achieved when the white stone or white elixir is purified further, becoming completely fixed and stable. This stage is symbolized by the phoenix rising from the ashes. Spiritually, it is the permanent awareness of the divine self and its dual nature. In later alchemical writing, after the fifteenth century, the four stages of the Great Work were made into three. The yellowing stage, which is called *citrinitas,* was combined with rubedo. This stage is represented by the sun and the dawn and is a stage preceding rubedo in the awakening to the divine nature.

Fly Agaric (*Amanita muscaria*): The Trickster and the Shaman

The fly agaric mushroom is one of the oldest plants to have been used by humankind for its entheogenic properties. The sacred mushroom cult, its own spiritual tradition, was built up around this mushroom. Its red cap with white spots is also one of the most recognizable symbols in the world. It has been called soma, little red man, magic mushroom, and amrita. This mushroom was introduced to Europe by Laplanders or Sami, the first native people of northern Europe. The

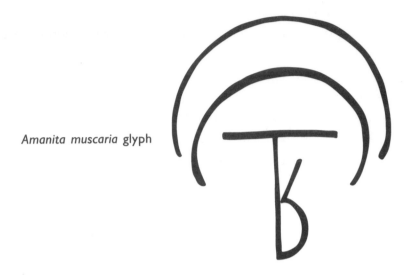

Amanita muscaria glyph

Sami were known for their sorcery, among other things. The Koryak and Kamchadaland, Finno-Ugrian tribes of western Siberia, were the first to use *Amanita muscaria*. The mushroom is thought by some to have been the source of the trance-like rage of the berserkers, fierce Norse warriors of northern Europe.

The Siberian Koryak attributed the creation of the mushrooms or *wa'paq* spirits to the deity Vahiyinin. According to the tale, the trickster Big Raven found these spirits so useful that he allowed them to remain on Earth and teach humans (Maestas 2007, 160). In the lore of the Northern Tradition, fly agaric is called *rabensbrot* (raven's bread) and was eaten by Odin's two ravens. It is closely associated with Odin, its spirit taking on a similar appearance. It was known by the ancient world to bring gifts of divination, healing, vitality, and open communication to the otherworld. It is intimately associated with elves, fairies, and nature spirits.

An ancient plant spirit, the fly agaric has many rules and customs that it expects to be observed by those who would seek its power. It is a traditional ritual entheogen and shamanic ally, allowing the user to travel between the worlds and see the complex web that weaves together life and death. The Latin root of *muscaria* is *musca,* meaning "to fly"

(Maestas 2007, 161). As a journeying ally, *Amanita muscaria* allows the user to ascend to both the heights and the depths of the world tree to meet the gods and seek out shades of the dead. It allows one to seek the cycle of death, giving insight into the process between death and rebirth.

Amanita muscaria can be found growing in the wild throughout the Northern Hemisphere after heavy rain, during the spring and fall. It also grows in temperate areas of the Eastern and Western Hemispheres, preferring the coniferous forests of pine, as well as birch and other hardwoods, forming a symbiotic relationship with these trees that connects the energies of the upper and lower realms. It has been used in the New World since before its colonization by Europeans. It can be found in parts of Canada and the United States, particularly the Pacific Northwest and the Great Lakes Region. The Ojibway of the Great Lakes Region and tribes of the Pacific Northwest all partook of this sacrament and recognized its spiritual power.

The characteristic spotted caps can reach a diameter larger than a human hand or be smaller than an inch in diameter. They range in color from red orange to light brown and gold. There are other varieties of *Amanita* that are extremely poisonous, such as *A. phalloides*, the appropriately named death cap mushroom. These other varieties look similar but are often brown, yellow, or white. There are some safe varieties of *A. muscaria* growing in North America that have a golden color, but proper identification is of the utmost importance.

Fly Agaric Dosages and Preparation

Fly agaric, or *Amanita muscaria,* has been used in traditional medicine to treat snakebites, fever, and epilepsy. It has pain-relieving and muscle-relaxing properties when applied topically. It also has a pronounced effect on the nervous system and has been used to treat anxiety, depression, and nerve pain.

Amanita muscaria contains the alkaloids muscimole, muscarine, choline, acetylcholine, macaridine, muscazone, and ibotenic acid. Muscimole is not actually present in the fresh mushroom but is converted from ibotenic acid during the drying process. Drying the mushrooms makes them more effective and reduces the amount of ibotenic acid, which is responsible for uncomfortable side effects such as nausea. Both ibotenic acid and muscimole are the main psychoactive ingredients in fly agaric. Muscarine is a tropane alkaloid present in small amounts; although this alkaloid is poisonous, most of it evaporates when the mushroom is dried (Miller 1983, 81). These components present an interesting balance between poison and spiritual food, which is often the case with these plants. There have been no deaths linked to the use of *Amanita muscaria* mushrooms, but the same cannot be said for its poisonous relatives. This is why it is very important to be certain you have identified the correct fungi.

Muscimol behaves atypically compared to other psychedelics. It activates the brain's receptors for GABA, the brain's primary inhibitory neurotransmitter, which contributes to its psychoactive effects. Some of the physiological effects experienced with *Amanita muscaria* are physical euphoria, color enhancement, disconnection from surroundings, vivid dreams, and a sense of interconnectedness. Ibotenic acid acts on the central nervous system and causes lethargy, drowsiness, drunkenness, heaviness in the body, muscle relaxation, and flushed red skin. Amanita experiences are described as both heaven and hell.

While the correct dosage will open the gates of perception, the wrong dosage will result in uncomfortable side effects. Smaller doses are compared to alcohol intoxication, and larger doses are psychoactive. It is difficult to determine a starting dose because the effects differ widely from one individual to another. A good rule of thumb is to start small, monitor the effects, and work your way up. Fly agaric can be added to smoking blends and is often combined with cannabis and nightshades, such as henbane, datura, and belladonna. This combination has synergistic effects, curbing some of the unwanted side effects associated with both botanicals. The dried mushrooms can be eaten by themselves or made into an alcohol extract or oil infusion. These can be taken in microdoses to benefit from the subtle vibrational effects the mushroom has to offer. Generally, a microdose is considered one-tenth a regular dose. While everyone is going to be different, 1 to 3 grams is going to have noticeable effects and is generally a good starting range. To give an idea of the strength of the tincture, it would take 30 ml of tincture to consume the equivalent of 3 grams.

Fly Agaric (*Amanita muscaria*) Tincture

- 25 g dried *Amanita muscaria* caps
- 250 ml vodka

Add the fly agaric and vodka to a mason jar. Allow to infuse for two to four weeks, shaking regularly. When complete, strain and discard the caps. This tincture is a 1:10 ratio, which is a good concentration for microdosing and enjoying the subtler medicinal effects of this fungus. The tincture can be taken by putting a few drops directly under the tongue and letting it sit there for around thirty seconds. The tincture and the oil (see below) can also be applied topically; they are said to have analgesic and anxiolytic properties. One thing to remember when ingesting *Amanita muscaria* is to avoid consuming any carbonated beverages. The carbon dioxide reverts the muscimol back to ibotenic acid and can make you sick.

To make the oil, you can use the same 1:10 ratio that we used in the tincture or a 1:5 ratio. Before covering the mushrooms with oil, you will want to powder them using a coffee grinder or mortar and pestle. Powdering the material exposes more surface area and enhances extraction. You can heat the oil and powder in a slow cooker or double boiler for four to six hours or allow them to infuse naturally. You don't have to strain the oil as the chemicals in the mushroom powder can be absorbed when in direct contact with the skin. This makes a great anointing oil for shamanic workings; apply to the temples and third eye.

Calamus (*Acorus calamus*): The Magical Stylus of Thoth

Calamus, or sweet flag, as it is also known, is a curious plant with historical references dating back to the time of the Old Testament and ancient Egypt. It is a well-known commanding and compelling ingredient in African American Hoodoo formulas and has been used as an aphrodisiac and stimulant. Its use in Hoodoo formulas is possibly based on the Old Testament. In a passage in Exodus 30:22–38, God gives Moses instructions to create a holy anointing oil. Calamus is one of the ingredients in this oil used to anoint the ark of the covenant and the tabernacle, where the most sacred and holy religious texts were kept. Individuals also applied the ointment to themselves before entering the tabernacle, which would have had an empowering effect, rendering the wearer holy.

The root of the plant is the part used in the creation of coercive formulas, often paired with licorice root, another commanding herb. This combination forms the basis of many compelling formulas of mastery, to which other herbs may be added to determine the type of influence one wishes to have. The root is powdered before being added to a condition oil (a spell or ritual oil). Like many other herbs with commanding properties, calamus may also be used to strengthen and bind spells. Following with the theme of magical catalysts, calamus brings a forceful will to whatever it is added to. Through the power of the written word, one can create change like the gods. The calamus reed along with ritually prepared inks allows the scribe to infuse his or her will onto the page.

The plant itself is a tall reedy plant that grows along streams and ponds among the cattails. It has a horizontally growing root that can reach up to five feet long. The root contains the majority of the plant's essential oils and active ingredients, which are collected for their ritual and medicinal uses. The root is prized for its chemical components, which have been used traditionally by tribal peoples for millennia. The chemicals within calamus can be taken in small amounts when a stimulating effect is desired. It is particularly beneficial for fasting and during long, arduous journeys. Indigenous people would chew on the root when out in the wilderness. Larger amounts would be used for their psychoactive properties, along with other ingredients in recipes for shamanic journeying (Miller 1983, 57).

Calamus root can be used as an incense for the illuminating,

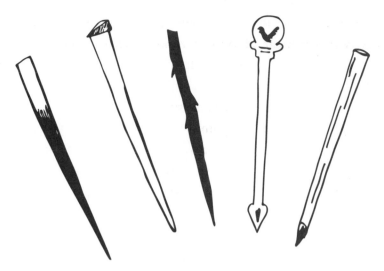

Sacred woods can be employed as writing utensils in spellcraft by charring one end and writing or drawing in its ash. This is a useful technique for cursing, banishing, and warding due to the properties of ash itself.

strengthening, and stimulating effects it has on the mind. It can be burned during meditation and ritual to increase concentration. The root contains high concentrations of essential oils. Its psychoactive properties are attributed to the presence of asarone. Interestingly, calamus contains safrole, which occurs also in sassafras and is involved in the synthesis of MDMA. The essential oil has tonic effects and pharmacologically acts similarly to papaverine derived from the poppy. It is unlikely that calamus is actually psychoactive or hallucinogenic; it doesn't appear to have any psychoactive chemicals. But with its aphrodisiac, strengthening, and stimulating properties, it does have some promising ritual uses as a kind of excitatory entheogen.

Parsley (*P. crispum* var *neapolitanum*): The Green Devil

Parsley, a common garnish and unassuming plant, once had a sinister reputation. Also called the devil's weed, parsley's diabolical and dark associations go back as far as ancient Greece, where it was a symbol of death used to decorated tombs. It was said to have sprung from the blood of Archemorus, a son of the Nemean king Lycurgus and Eurydice, whose name meant "forerunner of death." Parsley was also used as a garden border or hedge plant along with rue.

There are many intriguing bits of lore surrounding parsley and a diverse set of taboos regarding its use and planting. Parsley has a reputation in the English countryside as a plant of bad luck and ill omen, with superstitions varying from place to place. Parsley has a slow and irregular germination rate. Since it lies in the ground a long time before germinating, it was said to go down to the devil and back three to nine times, depending on the region, before sprouting. Those that didn't sprout, the devil kept for himself. There were taboos around the planting or transplanting of parsley, and several practices were devised to mitigate its baneful influence. As such, parsley could only be planted by a woman while church bells were ringing or on Good Friday.

It can be used to connect to the trickster spirits of the green realm—the green devil or adversarial spirit of nature, the lord of the hunt and wandering spirit of the wildwood. Parsley is used in formulas for sending out one's spirit into the night and to increase one's cunning and knowledge of the spirit world. It was often included as an ingredient in recipes for medieval flying ointments, sometimes listed as *silium,* from *Petroselium,* the medieval Latin genus name for the plant, a Latinized form of the Greek word *petroselinon,* meaning "rock celery." Interestingly, its leaves, flowers, and root resemble those of poison hemlock, also known as fool's parsley or poison parsley. Much of the sinister lore connected to parsley may be due to this resemblance, a connection that has been forged over centuries. Parsley was known to counteract poisons, which is thought to be the origin for its continued use as a garnish. This may also be connected to parsley's ability to counteract the smell of garlic on one's breath.

Lady's Mantle (*Alchemilla vulgaris*): The Little Alchemist

Lady's mantle is not poisonous or psychoactive, but it is a magical cata-lyst and an ally to the herbalist, alchemist, and wort cunner. The plants known as magical catalysts have an affinity for the work of the magician and alchemist, in part due to their history, their correspondence with other occult forces, and the lore and traditions that have accumulated around them. The plants within this Mercurian category make power-ful allies and willing teachers for the exploration of alchemy and the art of potion making. The planetary correspondences of these plants are often contradictory and difficult to pin down, which is a characteristic of the trickster spirit. Their apparent connection to the Great Work falls within the realm of Mercury, the thrice great alchemist.

Lady's mantle, the little alchemist, is a patron plant of both herbal-ists and alchemists and is a perfect example of this category of plants. Its name refers to the shape of the plant's leaves, which unfold like little cloaks. It is a common plant in the Northern Hemisphere and is his-torically connected to the goddess Freya and fairy lore in Europe. The plant corresponds to the elements earth and water, which attests to her feminine energy. She can help us unlock the secrets of nature through herbal alchemy and plant magic, helping us connect with the nurturing power of Mother Earth. She helps one attune with one's own earthy feminine side.

As an herb of glamour and enchantment, the plant itself and the dew that collects in her leaves were used for their enchanting effects and in beautification rituals, often as a face wash to impart other-worldly allure. Lady's mantle is appropriately a powerful women's herb, under the rule of Venus. Its medicinal properties as a women's tonic have a number of beneficial uses. The connections with beauty, feminine mystique, and love are all due to the plant's correspondence with the goddess of love. The plant has a long history of use in love philters and potions. All parts of the plant may be dried and powdered to create a base for other formulas, reflecting her role as a vehicle for magical preparations.

Alchemilla vulgaris was well known to medieval alchemists. Although not a baneful herb, her efficacy as a plant ally has earned her a place among magical catalysts. Alchemists recognized the powerful potential of this plant, making it the basis for many of their formulas. Medieval alchemists, who called her stellaria, used her celestial waters. The sacred liquid found in her leaves had properties of transmutation that were desirable for the Great Work. Stellaria brings celestial and lunar power to formulas, her power further enhanced when the plant is collected according to the phases of the moon.

Dew, a sacred condensation and thought to be the nectar of the moon, appeared overnight on the plant and would be gathered the next day. To collect the dew, cotton cheesecloth was draped over the plant at night, and after the cloth absorbed this nocturnal virtue, the sacred water was wrung from the cloth and used in alchemical preparations, lustral waters, and glamorizing washes. Small amounts of dew collected directly from the plant's cup-shaped leaves would also be used. Drinking from these natural vessels was said to enchant the aura, and small amounts were used to wash the eyes for second sight and looking beyond the veil.

The dew, collected before sunrise, was an important ingredient in alchemical operations. A universal magical potentiator, the dew can be tinctured with plant material for later use in other preparations. The potential applications for such a universal tool are endless, and having a tincture of lady's mantle on hand is an asset for the alchemist and green witch. This arcane formula can be used as a magical activator and in rituals of transformation known as *altera et alteram*, which involve the creation of magical tools and objects through transmutation of their spiritual energies. The plant's properties of alchemical transformation are used in the transmigration of serpent power or witch fire from the dragon lines of Earth through the sorcerer and into the desired vessel.

As a plant spirit familiar, lady's mantle helps those on the Crooked

Path connect with other plant spirits and teaches us their hidden virtues. She can also help with connecting with the darker spirits of the plant realm, providing her own protection and insight when dealing with these more dangerous allies, acting as an emissary.

꙰

Greater Periwinkle (*Vinca major*): The Sorcerer's Violet

Greater periwinkle, also known as myrtle and the sorcerer's violet, finds its way into the collection of magical allies due to its many uses in folk magic during the Middle Ages. This plant seems to have more uses in magic and enchantment than it does in everyday applications. Greater periwinkle is a plant of the fairy realm, growing along the wayside and on the forest floor, quickly spreading its early-blooming violet flowers. *Vinca major* is another five-petaled plant, the number of Venus and a number connected to plants used in magic, including many of the visionary plants. Five-petaled plants, among them the nightshade family, act as gateways, like the pentagram, which they resemble.

Greater periwinkle is the perfect plant to collect for Beltane to celebrate the beauty and new life of spring. Its astringent, antiseptic, and deodorant properties were used in baths of beautification. The leaves and flowers were collected and used in infusions and lustral waters for toning and firming the skin and imparting a health glow to the skin and an otherworldly allure. The plant can also be used in scrying vessels for peering into the otherworld.

This plant is attractive to nature spirits in general and can be used as an offering for woodland spirits, plant allies, and elemental entities. *Vinca major* is particularly associated with the fairy realm and is used in rituals to connect with these energies. It also has connections to the lunar energy of the moon, and when used during full moon divination rituals, it yields powerful results. Medieval lore suggests that it be gathered on the days numerically associated with the moon—the first, ninth, eleventh, or thirteenth days of the lunar cycle. It is an herb of cleansing and purification, and its protective properties are used to expel fear, clarify situations, and promote groundedness and strength.

Sorcerer's violet has been used in charms to protect against dog bites and snake poison and to exorcise evil spirits. It was historically used in binding and in coercive love spells and often appears in medieval love formulas for drawing and binding two people together.

> *I pray thee, vinca pervinca, thee that art to be had for thy many useful qualitites, that thou come to me glad-blossoming with thine mainfulness, that thou outfit me so that I be shielded and ever prosperous and undamaged by poison and water.*
>
> APULEIUS, *HERBARIUM*, 1480

Wolfsbane (*Aconitum* spp.): High Queen of Poisons

A. napellus, A. carmichaeli, A. foresteri, A. vulparia, and *A. lycotonum* are just a few of the varieties in this large group of plants. These plants belong to the Ranunculaceae family with 150 other species in this genus. Aconite or wolfsbane, as it is commonly called, is known for being the most poisonous plant genus in Europe, having a large body of myth and lore associated with it. Wolfsbane and monkshood are similar plants, and the names are often used interchangeably to describe all aconites. From a magical perspective, they are so similar that they can be used interchangeably. Some herbalists claim that *A. lycotonum,* with its white and yellow flowers, is the one old herbals refer to when mentioning wolfsbane. The blue and purple variety, *A. napellus,* was commonly grown in apothecary gardens in medieval monasteries and is referred to as monkshood—appropriate for its resemblance to the hooded monks who grew this plant.

The plant is sacred to several spirits with connections to magic and the Poison Path. It was once the most important of magical plants of a poisonous nature because it was used to combat were-wolves. It was historically referred to as *hecateis,* named after Hecate, for whom the plant was sacred, having grown from the saliva spilled by her three-headed dog Cerberus, guardian of the gates to the under-world. Cerberus served as Hecate's protector in the same way that this plant protects its allies. Wolfsbane has a strong affinity with Hecatean magic; lore about this plant mentions it being used by Hecate and her descendants. In her aspect as Hecate Lycania, she is patron of were-wolves and shape-shifters and can be invoked for her aid in the arts of shape-shifting. Wolfsbane is also associated with Apollo and the witch Medea.

Monkshood also has a prominent place in the magical pharma-copeia of the Northern Tradition. It was called *thüng* by the Anglo-Saxons, an Old English term for any extremely poisonous plant. In Norse mythology, it is known as Odin's helm, *trollhat* (Norse trollscap), and *Venuswagon* and is connected to Odin and the goddess Hel.

Interestingly, regarding lycanthropy—the supernatural transforma-tion of a person into a wolf or the delusion of being a wolf—symptoms of this poison have been described as tingling and creepy-crawly sensa-tions (Grieve 1971), which could be compared to moving through the air or the feeling of having fur or feathers. It also has a numbing effect, which would make one more tolerant to pain. It may have contrib-uted to some of the legends of lycanthropy. Some tales suggest that the Scythians may have used wolfsbane in preparation for shape-shifting (Rätsch 2005, 35). Wolfsbane was said to have been used in battle by Germanic berserkers, who were known for their battle rage. Its use was likely talismanic considering the symptoms of respiratory and cardiac suppression if ingested. The Germanic berserkers and Scythians were thought of as shape-shifters who took on the qualities of the wolf. As a plant used in warfare wolfsbane was sacred also to gods of war like Tyr/Thor and was called Thor's helmet. It was also used to create poison-tipped arrows for killing both men and wolves, which is where it earned the name *wolfsbane.* The toxic arrows would poison not only their vic-tims but anyone who tried to remove the arrows as well.

In antiquity this plant was mentioned by Pliny the Elder in *Natural History,* where the plant is designated as "the most prompt of all poisons." The first recorded story mentioning aconite was told by Homer and later Ovid in *Metamorphoses.* Mythology mentions Medea, the sorceress, attempting to poison Theseus with aconite. The goddess Athena used the magical plant to turn Arachne into a spider, further evidence of its shape-shifting capabilities.

Using Wolfsbane in Magical Practice

This sinister plant has long ago earned its place in the witch's garden, and the name *queen of poisons* is most appropriate for such a deadly plant. Wolfsbane holds an undeniable aura of magic and mystery combined with a sense of danger and fear regarding its ability to kill with ease. This is like the dual nature of the witch, both alluring and deadly at the same time. It is an herb of empowerment for the shapeshifter and lycanthrope, helping them master their skills. It also aids in aspecting with animal familiars in an attempt to integrate their

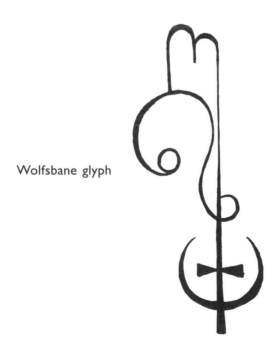

Wolfsbane glyph

wild nature. It is perfect for soul flight or hag riding and traveling in bestial forms. It helps the traveler maintain their animal body when in the astral realm.

Wolfsbane is an herb of chthonic Mercury and telluric fire, the mysterious dragon energy of Earth itself. It aids in the underworld journey, when one travels deep into the hidden places of the world to return with arcane knowledge. It protects one from spiritual parasites when journeying to realms of shadow, such as the realms of Hel or Jotunheim of the Norse tradition.

The tiny and numerous seeds of the plant along with its delicate leaves are characteristic of its Mercurian correspondence. The correlation between the axis mundi and the tall stem of this plant is another characteristic of its role as a journeying ally. Of course, the toxic and sinister nature of this plant is Saturnian, speaking to the dark side of Mercury. Its use in battle and as a chemical weapon also give it a Martian association to which Saturn is the higher octave. Just like the poisoned arrow, this plant is useful for magical sendings of spell and spirit, ensuring they reach their target. Using this plant as an addition to hexing formulas is like putting the poison on the head of an already deadly arrow, adding an especially malevolent quality.

Wolfsbane is most effectively used as an anointing oil for ritual tools and relics used for shamanic journeying. The soft violet flowers of monkshood are a sight to behold when its stalks are placed upon the altar. It has traditionally been used to empower and consecrate ritual objects, especially magical weapons. For example, anointing a ritual blade would render it effective against harmful spirits and astral parasites, facilitating their removal.

Although aconite is an extremely dangerous herb in the wrong hands, it is also very protective to those who do not offend its spirit by using it recklessly. Like many of the baneful herbs, it protects by stealth and subterfuge, allowing one to move about unnoticed.

Wolfsbane is used in dark moon rituals and rituals honoring the goddess Hecate. It can be used to call upon the ancient power of the Thessalian witches, who were associated with the goddess. According to lore, the witches of Thessaly, who were well known in the ancient world, specialized in the magical arts, including the use of aphrodisiacs and anaphrodisiacs. They provided birth control and helped terminate unwanted pregnancy. They specialized in the venefic and venereal arts, creating elixirs using the plants of Hecate's garden for spirit travel, longevity, and restoration. Wolfsbane was said to have been used by the Thessalian witches in their ointments.

Wolfsbane Dosages and Preparation

The toxic nature of this plant makes it dangerous to use in incense blends, formulas meant for ingestion, and ointments meant for topical application. The alkaloids in wolfsbane slow the heart rate and breathing. Liquid vessels or philters (powders) are a safer way of working with this plant, incorporating it into formulas not intended for ingestion. However, direct contact with the plant and its preparations can result in irritation. I have personally experimented with small amounts of the leaves infused in oil and have applied the oil topically to relieve pain due to the numbing effect it has on the nervous system. I recommend using dry plant material since the toxicity is greatly reduced. However, the nightshades are just as effective and less risky. Aconite is best for acute pain; I wouldn't recommend using aconite long term for chronic pain.

Traditionally, wolfsbane has been used in topical treatments, including liniments and ointments for neuralgia and lower back pain. Properly prepared tinctures were employed to reduce the heart rate at the onset of a fever and to reduce inflammation, taking up to five drops per day. The plant is used in traditional Chinese medicine; typically the root is used, and its alkaloid content diminishes greatly once dried. Aconite has been used in combination with belladonna to treat nerve pain, sciatica, rheumatism, colds, and migraine. It is used homeopathically for nervous disorders. Using aconite in these ways should be done only under the guidance of an experienced herbalist, however; just 0.2 mg of pure aconitine can produce toxic symptoms, such as slowed heart rate and respiration.

All parts of the plant contain the alkaloid aconitine, which is a potent neurotoxin and cardiotoxin. It acts on voltage-sensitive sodium channels in the cell membrane, causing major disruption. This affects the nerves, muscles, and myocardium. The highest concentration of alkaloids is found in the root (0.3–2.0 percent) and fresh seeds, with lower amounts in the leaves and stems. The overall alkaloid content increases during the growing season and is highest when the plant is in flower (June–July). The plant is most dangerous when it is fresh, the alkaloid content being reduced in dry plant material. I have personally handled fresh wolfsbane with no negative effects; however, if the juice gets on the skin, especially near an open cut, the body can absorb the toxins. Just 5 ml of juice from the plant is enough to kill an adult.

※

Wild Lettuce (*Lactuca virosa*): Food for the Dead

This unassuming plant, similar in appearance to its relative the dandelion and just as common in some areas, has been used since ancient times as an offering to the dead and the deities of the ancestral underworld. *Lactuca virosa* has a tall stalk with elongated leaves, yellow flowers, and feathery seeds. It is easily confused with other plants in the genus such as *Lactuca serriola,* which is similar in appearance and has many properties in common with wild lettuce, also known as prickly lettuce. The chemical compounds found in the plant are used to induce trance, providing a vehicle for visionary travel and prophetic dreams.

This plant was known in the ancient world for its narcotic and sedative effects, which are similar to those of the poppy. Like the poppy, it exudes a milky latex when cut. *Lactuca* means "milky extract," and *virosa* means "toxic." It is commonly called opium lettuce for its pain-relieving effects and can be smoked or applied topically, as well as ingested in tincture form. It is the dried milk sap, known as *lactuarium,* that is collected from the plant and used for this purpose. Somniferous, sleep-inducing plants like this relate to the nocturnal spirits of sleep and dreams; in Greek mythology they were Morpheus and Hypnos and were thought to be the children of either Hecate or the primordial goddess of the night, Nyx.

In this aspect, wild lettuce can be used for nocturnal workings seeking to utilize the subtle powers of the night and its shape-shifting inhabitants. It is related to the workings of the dark moon and can be used for bindings sent through dreams and to cause confusion in the waking mind.

As a dream-inducing and journeying plant, wild lettuce is safer to use than some of the more toxic plants of the nightshade family. However, wild lettuce does contain trace amounts of hyoscyamine, which is an alkaloid found in henbane. Its effects are anticonvulsant, hypnotic, sedative, diuretic, and laxative.

The sap would be collected as it was by Native Americans by cutting off the flower head and allowing the liquid to run out. It would then be dried and powdered before being used in smoking blends for visions and shamanic rituals. Lactuarium is not easily powdered, and it is only slightly soluble in boiling water. The leaves and root were also collected and dried to be used in these smoking blends. The chemicals in the plant material induce brain activity that is conducive to dreaming, making dreams more vivid and memorable. In large amounts, it results in toxicity; symptoms include mydriasis and photophobia, in addition to cardiovascular and respiratory difficulty. Its poisoning effects are similar to those of other plants that contain tropane-alkaloids, although larger amounts of this plant would be required.

Blood of the Gods

This plant is touched by the spirit of Saturn but is also Mercurian in nature, showing us again the dark side of Mercury, who travels to the underworld, leading newly deceased souls to their resting place. In this aspect, the messenger spirit helps us connect us with the ancestors and primal spirits of nature living within Earth. In Mercury's celestial aspect, he ascends to the upper spheres where the gods and other beings of light exist.

In this guise he is the trickster, the dark woodland spirit, who has a sinister side when it comes to working with humans. He is the adversary in nature who tests us through initiation and tribulation to determine if we are worthy of his secret knowledge.

Slain Gods, Light Bringers, and Punishment

Ancient Greek manuscripts refer to *Lactuca virosa* as Titan's blood, which speaks of this plant's divine status. The Titans were led by Kronos, who was equated with the Roman deity Saturn, an amalgam of two primal indigenous deities known for teaching humankind how to reap the bounty of the Earth through agriculture. In this form, he has more in common with the Mercurian horned god of nature, honored by witches and pagans alike, bringing the gifts of civilization as seen in the Luciferian and Promethean archetypal mythos. Like the other gods who were punished for gifting humankind with the arts and crafts of civilization and the power of fire, Saturn/Kronos was given a more negative connotation over time.

Wild lettuce is also connected to the goddess Aphrodite through the death of her lover Adonis. When slain, he was laid on a bed of wild lettuce. In some versions of the story, he was slain by a wild boar among the plant. After his death, wild lettuce became associated with the death of love or impotency and was used as an anaphrodisiac. The myth of Aphrodite and Adonis is based on the earlier Sumerian myth of Ishtar/Inanna and Tammuz/Dumuzid. Tammuz was an early god of vegetation and shepherding, playing the role of the slain god in witchcraft mythos.

As previously mentioned, wild lettuce was referred to as Titan's blood, and the oozing lactuarium coming from breaks in the plant, resembling blood dripping from a wound, gives us some powerful imagery and mythology to work with. Ichor was the all-powerful blood of the gods and was spilled by Prometheus as part of his punishment from Zeus for bringing fire to early man. This fire taken from the gods and given to man can be equaled to Luciferian gnosis, the knowledge given to man by the serpent. The fallen angels that taught the daughters of man the magical arts and how to work with herbs left a legacy in the concept of witch-blood or the mark of Cain, which is an esoteric concept of a spiritual bloodline connecting all witches and practitioners of the magical arts.

Another Promethean/Mercurian deity, Loki, was punished by the gods for the death of Baldr. Part of his punishment was to have the venom of a snake drip over him for eternity. His loyal wife, Sigyn, catches the poison in a vessel. When the vessel is full, she must remove it to empty it, and only then does the poison fall on Loki. The poison-filled vessel is a symbolic representation of the Poison Path.

⚘

Centaury (*Centaurium erythraea*): Chiron, the Wounded Healer

Centaury is a curious little herb, rustic and simple in appearance, blending in with other plants within the medicinal apothecary garden. It is not a baneful herb, but it is a patron herb of herbalists and anyone that works with plants. Centaury is named after Chiron (Kheiron), the eldest and wisest of the race of centaurs. Half-man, half-horse humanoid creatures, centaurs were known for their wisdom and also for their ambivalence and animosity toward humankind.

Some of the myths associated with Chiron tell us that Kronos was his father, yet another Saturnian connection. In his original form as an agricultural god, Chiron gained his wisdom of plants from his father and through him was also marked as "other." It was said that he lived in Thessaly at the foot of a mountain. Thessaly was known as a place of magic and mystery and was also home to the famous witches of the time.

> *The science of herbs and drugs was discovered by*
> *Chiron, the son of Saturnus and Philyra.*
> PLINY THE ELDER, *NATURAL HISTORY*, BOOK 7

Astrologically, the small planetoid Chiron has some interesting connections based on its relationship with its planetary neighbors. This planetoid—not to be confused with Charon, Pluto's moon, which is named after the ferryman on the River Styx—has an extremely eccentric orbit. Chiron orbits between Saturn and Neptune, placing it in an interesting position between the inner and outer solar system. In this space, Chiron acts as a sort of shadow counterpart to Mercury, as the intermediary between the personal realm of the inner solar system and the shadowy depths of the collective consciousness represented by the outer planets.

Gall of the Earth, Fel Wort, Fel Terrae

As a plant well known for its applications in magic and ritual herb craft, centaury gained many of its fantastic associations with the arcane in the Middle Ages. It was commonly grown in medieval apothecary gardens for its medicinal properties. These gardens were also home to many of the plants that became connected to magical practices. This plant is mentioned in *Le Petit Albert,* a magical grimoire, as one of fifteen sacred herbs of the ancients.

The grimoire mentions the plant's use in magical lamps, combined with other botanical materials known for their magical properties. Centaury, the grimoire tells us, can be used in the oil of the lamp as a central focal point to the rites of the medieval witches' sabbat, said to "make all who compass about it believe themselves to be witches." It brings the bearer a magical aura of wisdom and knowledge, influencing the way the bearer is perceived by others.

In the myths of Chiron the centaur, he was responsible for teaching many individuals the medicinal properties of plants, most notably the physician Asclepius, who became a patron of healers and medicine. In practice, the plant can be used to connect with the spirit of its namesake when learning about medicinal herbalism and natural healing. It makes a powerful ally for green witches, wort cunners, and root workers whose practice is based in the green arts. Like many five-petaled plants, centaury has become a patron ally of the magical arts, encompassing the working of both balms and banes. Centaury's essence is healing and nourishing to the spirit, emotions, and psyche. It is a plant for healing the healer and reminding those who serve others to take care of themselves as well.

As a flower essence, it can be used by energy workers, intuitive healers, and spiritual advisers. Flower essences contain the energetic signature of the plant they are made from, extracted into distilled water while in the sunlight. These essences have profound effects on our mental, emotional, and spiritual bodies. Centaury flower essence is perfect for those who are newly developing their abilities. It keeps one uninfluenced by the energetic detritus of others, while maintaining one's own personal will and identity. It can be used for repelling anger, unwanted influence, and harmful energy, especially for those working as spiritual healers and those who are regularly exposed to stagnant or unhealthy energies in the environment. It restores vitality to the energy system of the healer, especially after clearing and cleansing a place of heavy malevolent energies. It can be included as part of one's own regimen for maintaining the health of one's own subtle bodies, which is especially useful for magical practitioners, keeping them empowered for the healing of others. It helps the healer maintain his or her own personal protection and energetic hygiene in the healer's line of work. Centaury is also useful after prolonged illness and intense healing sessions to revitalize the body and spirit.

In ritual the dried plant material can be used in incense to induce trance states and achieve deeper meditation, specifically when meditating on and connecting with the living Earth. Centaury connects us with the green writhing serpent fire of the natural world that enlivens all living things. As a tutelary herb and plant ally, centaury can be used as a magical catalyst, alone or mixed with other power-enhancing plants like lady's mantle, its female counterpart. The combination of both plants creates a powerful all-purpose formula for the green alchemist.

Chiron represents the wounded healer archetype: he gains his healing capacity through tribulation or initiation in which a part of himself is removed, destroyed, or changed. The wounded healer is incapacitated in some way, causing him to discover his innate healing abilities, leaving behind something new. Centaury helps in the facilitation and integration of this experience.

✼

Enchanter's Nightshade (*Circaea lutetiana*): The Dread Goddess

Witch's grass, sorcerer of Paris, and great witch herb are some of the other names given to this wild-growing woodland plant, which has connections to sorcery via its namesake Circe. Daughter of Hecate, queen of the witches, Circe is well versed in the venefic arts of potion making and manipulative magic. A potent female figure, feared for her power, she was once known as the "dread goddess who walks with mortals."

The plant is not actually a nightshade but a member of the evening primrose family. It is native to the Northeast in North America, Europe, central Asia, and Siberia and grows in wooded areas and along pathways. The small white flowers have two petals and are the first indication of this plant's Saturnian connection to the underworld.

Due to this plant's connection to the ancient myths of the sorceress Circe and her reputation for powerful hexes and curses thrown upon her enemies, we can use this plant in a similar way, drawing on its connections forged through myth and spirit. The burrs that form on this plant can be used to one's advantage. They attach themselves to fur and clothing to help spread their seed over a wide area. The tendency of this plant to attach itself to others can be used in sympathetic magic when a long-lasting attachment of a spell is desired. Plants that spread their seeds in this way can also help us connect to the spirit of the wanderer, an archetype seen in the figures Odin and Cain, who through their wanderings discover great wisdom.

As a tutelary spirit sympathetic to witches, and female witches in particular, the "dread goddess" Circe is a fierce protectress of her kind. She will help with works of vengeance and swift justice, unafraid to use her power to turn her enemies into swine. Offensive workings, hexing, cursing, and crossing can all be aided by propitiating this goddess.

As a daughter of Hecate, Circe is well versed in herb craft, particularly the plant's magical applications. Having spent much time in the garden of Hecate, Circe has gained, under Hecate's tutelage, extensive knowledge about potion making and magical formulas. Call upon her especially during potion making to bless and empower philters, elixirs, and other botanical formulas.

SEEDS, PODS, AND SPORES: MESSENGERS OF THE PLANT KINGDOM

Plants ruled by Mercury generally have numerous small seeds, ensuring that they travel far and wide. Seeds contain all of the genetic information of a fully mature plant. They are the blueprint of the adult plant, a very Mercurian quality. Mercurian plants stimulate or calm the mind by acting on the nervous system. The plants are used for focus, motivation, and energy or for their calming, contemplative, and meditative effects. They are characterized by their effects on the brain and nervous system.

Seeds have been used traditionally for the opposite effects—to cause confusion or to induce obsessive-compulsive behavior. Mustard seeds used to be sprinkled outside the home because it was believed that vampires had to count all of the seeds before they could enter, and they wouldn't be able to do so before sunrise. Poppy seeds are used in hexes to cause confusion. Here is a list of seeds and their magical uses.

Black cumin seeds (*Nigella sativa*): These seeds are used in glamour magic, shape-shifting spells, and memory spells and can be employed to cause forgetfulness. Also called blessing seeds, they have a sinister quality and can be used in rituals for magical warfare. Black cumin seeds can made into an oil used as a tonic to decalcify the pineal gland and open the third eye.

Black mustard seeds (*Brassica nigra*): These tiny seeds are known for their use in bringing confusion to enemies. They have been used historically to protect against witches, vampires, and evil spirits. They cause scattered thought and broken speech. When used to keep away unwanted persons, they are sprinkled around the area while walking backward.

Celery seeds (*Apium graveolens*): Like many Mercurian seeds, celery seeds increase clarity, insight, and mental powers. They can be used to feed tarot cards and other divination tools and to enhance psychic ability.

Dill seeds (*Anethum graveolens*): The dill plant produces a multitude of seeds, which is characteristic of a Mercurian plant. Thus, it is an herb of multiplication and increase. It can be used in workings for knowledge and creative inspiration and for acquiring information and bringing out the truth. It is a plant of many thoughts. Medicinally, it calms anxiety and panic, bringing clarity to the anxious mind. Its scent helps us focus. It was allegedly used in medieval magic to rob witches of their will.

Fennel seeds (*Foeniculum vulgare*): Fennel is a classical witching herb and, when taken under the tongue, can be used to add power to speech, making the speaker eloquent and sweet of tongue. It gives extra force to the spoken word, helping to carry it over long distances. It can be use in spells of countermagic. Fennel is often included in incense recipes for summoning spirits, giving them speech. Prometheus was said to have carried fire down from Mount Olympus on a great fennel stalk. Fennel is also one of the ingredients in the Anglo-Saxon Nine Herbs Prayer.

Henbane seeds (*Hyoscyamus niger*): Although the entire plant has many uses for the magical practitioner, henbane seeds in particular are known for their power to open the gateways to those who would travel to the upper and lower realms. The seeds are given as offerings to the dead and used as an ingredient in incense to produce a trance-inducing smoke, inhaled for its hypnotic effect. The seeds are known for the consistency of their chemical composition, being more predictable and less intense than other alkaloid-containing plants.

Poppy seeds (*Papaver* spp.): Poppies have a long history of use in both magic and medicine and have been used for their ability to bring calm, ease pain, and induce sleep. They were thought to be included in witches' flying ointments to counter some of the adverse effects of deadly nightshade and also to be an antidote for its poison. Poppies are under the domain of the moon and nocturnal deities, such as Nyx, Morpheus, and Hypnos. (Read more about this Venusian herb in chapter 6.)

Mercury is the ruler of communication; it brings charisma and eloquence. It is a mental planet, ruling the mind and nervous system. Mercurian energy helps us get our message out into the world and charm others in the process. Using the symbolic association of "planting a seed," we can create a formula to influence the mind of another person. Seeds contain infinite potential, and we can use that potential to influence the way others perceive reality.

Seeds can be used to send glamours or to plant ideas in people's minds. This can be achieved by sending dreams or projecting an image into the target's mind. By using glamour magic in this way, you are sending an image of what you want an individual to perceive. The formula, once completed, can be worn as a charm to affect one's aura and influence those around one. Or it can be incorporated into a poppet to affect the body and behavior of a specific person or used with a skull to affect the mind. The following formula contains herbs associated with eloquence, manipulation, and mental discord.

✧✦✧

Seeds of Discord Powder

- 🌱 Ashes of rosemary (*Rosmarinus officinalis*): for forgetfulness
- 🌱 Black cumin or blessing seeds (*Nigella sativa*): for glamour and shape-shifting
- 🌱 Celery seeds (*Apium graveolens*): to distract
- 🌱 Datura seeds (*Datura stramonium*): to control the will of another and his or her perception of reality
- 🌱 Grains of paradise (*Aframomum melegueta*): to command and compel
- 🌱 Poppy seeds (*Papaver* spp.): for confusion and a sense of complacency

🤙 **Wolfsbane seeds (*Aconitum lycoctonum*): for invisibility and shape-shifting**

The seeds are ground to a powder along with the ashes while focusing on the individual and your intent. Spoken charms may be added, and the formula is sprinkled in a ritual manner or worn in a vial around the neck to influence those in direct proximity.

MERCURIAN ARTIFICE: ARCANE OBJECTS AND MAGICAL CATALYSTS

The following elements and objects are imbued with Mercurian energy and have various uses in rituals and magic making.

Snakeskins: The skin of a serpent is widely known for its protective properties and connection with shape-shifting, occult wisdom, and transformation. It will protect the sorcerer when traveling in spirit.

Hazel wood wands and bundles: This classical wood is used in magicians' wands. A hazel wand is used to connect with spirits, to open and close dimensional doorways, and for finding energy vortexes. Hazel twigs are used to create protective bundles used in healing rituals and to provide protection from many unseen forces. Small twigs are placed around the personal belongings of an individual and are tied together; this bundle is then wrapped in cloth with sacred herbs. The bundle is treated with utmost care. Healing incense can be used to smoke it, which can be incorporated into further ritual. Keep the bundle on the altar and tucked safely away in a box when not in use. (For more about hazel, see chapter 8.)

Quicksilver: Liquid mercury, the corresponding metal of the planet, is highly toxic. When mercury is ingested or contacts the skin, little is absorbed, usually not enough to be harmful. However, mercury gives off an invisible gas when spilled and is especially toxic if inhaled.

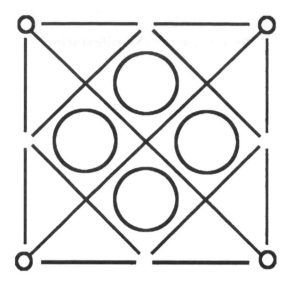

The seal of Mercury: Used to imbue talismans and charms with
the planetary powers of this celestial sphere. The seal itself can
also be carried as a talisman for its effects on eloquence, wisdom,
communication, mental clarity, and traveling.

(From Agrippa, *Three Books of Occult Philosophy*)

If worn in a glass vial around the neck, quicksilver can protect one
from malevolent entities. It can be used in the ritual circle without
the more disruptive qualities of iron.

Scrying stones: A crystal sphere or quartz point suspended between
the prongs of a stang serve as a focal point for scrying and inducing
trance. A stang is a two-pronged staff used in traditional witchcraft.
It is a masculine symbol, suggestive of the tines of a stag's antler.
Symbolic of the "Light Betwixt the Horns," the source of occult
illumination, it can be used for rituals that involve astral projection
or sending one's spirit across far distances. It can be placed on the
altar or stood at the periphery of the ritual circle, at the cardinal
point that corresponds to the working at hand.

Ancestral spirit bottle: A focal point for ancestral altars and necromantic empowerment, the bottle serves as a spirit vessel and anchor
for their manifestation.

⚘⚘

Spirit Vessel of Manifestation

- Salt
- Frankincense
- Henbane
- Mugwort
- Mullein
- Myrrh
- Wolfsbane flowers
- Wormwood
- 1 drop sorcerer's blood

Equal parts of the ingredients are layered in a consecrated vessel, which is then sealed with wax. A drop of one's own blood will add additional power, connecting with one's individual ancestry. Adorning the vessel with bones and other symbols of the dead adds to its symbolic power, while interring it in the ground, ideally a graveyard, enhances its connection with the other side. The bottle is kept on the ancestral altar after its preparation, and regular offerings of smoke and libation are made to it.

8

Other Magical Plants

Catalysts, Euphoriants, and Cleansers

*N*ot every plant associated with magic is a deadly poison. Many plants that have a rich body of magical lore associated with them have many uses in medicine and have amazing healing properties. Covered in this chapter are plants that are not closely associated with a particular planet but are well known for their affinity with spellcasters and magical practice. There are herbs for creating boundaries, hiding your workings, and discovering occult knowledge. Many of these herbs are magical catalysts or already have some association with magic and witchcraft, making them powerful allies for the green practitioner. Their unique properties and correspondences make them well suited for aiding the performance of magic rituals and ceremonies. Each of these plants has a unique quality that sets it apart from the usual protection, prosperity, and love magic.

PLANT CATALYSTS

Plants that seem to resonate with the magician's art are called *magical catalysts* because, in addition to their unique properties and application, they have a universal empowering effect, acting as potentiators when added to any formula. These plants often display two or more elemental or planetary attributes and have transformative effects, depending on the other plants that they are combined with.

Agrimony (*Agrimonia eupatoria*): Agrimony offers powerful protection from magic and dangerous spirits and is used in spells to cause sleep and to move about unnoticed. It returns negativity and seals it there, making it a beneficial herb for deflecting magical attack. It can be added to protection spells to reinforce them or used alone to create protective boundaries. It strengthens and fortifies the aura and one's natural defenses. (Agrimony is discussed further in chapter 5.)

Black horehound (*Ballota nigra*): This horehound prefers nitrogen-rich alkaline soils and grows in ruins, fallows, and hedges. It has a fetid odor that is moldy and musty and can be used to garner protection from land spirits.

Centaury (*Centaurium erythraea*): This patron plant of herbalists is named after the centaurs, half-man, half-horse beings who taught people the healing properties of herbs. It was used widely in magic in the Middle Ages. Centaury increases psychic ability, induces trance, and adds potency to herbal mixtures. As a plant ally, it aids the practitioner in learning the deeper secrets of the plant world. (Centaury is discussed further in chapter 7.)

Enchanter's nightshade (*Circaea lutetiana*): This plant, named after the famous sorceress Circe, adds power to enchantments, glamour magic, and coercive magic. It is a useful herb for invocations of witch goddesses and can be used for dark moon rituals and spells of transformation. It is a Mercurean plant, related to other nightshades only by name. (Enchanter's nightshade is discussed further in chapter 7.)

Oak galls or serpents' eggs: These round abnormal growths that occur on oak trees have long been considered to have magical properties. The galls are caused by wasps injecting their larvae into the tree's bark. They are used as magical catalysts and can be added to any mixture to increase its potency. They can also be used to create magical ink.

Skullcap (*Scutellaria lateriflora*): Medicinally, skullcap is used for its calmative and relaxing properties. Magically, it can be used to reveal hidden knowledge and made into an infusion to be taken after ritual as a restorative. It also is useful before meditation or divination.

Slippery elm (*Ulmus rubra*): Known for its use in spells to stop gossip, slippery elm can also be used to make one's magic untraceable and in spells to cause someone to tell the truth or divulge secrets. For its cloaking effects, it is strewn about the altar.

Thorn apple (*Datura stramonium*): One of the famous plants of the nightshade family, thorn apple is intimately associated with witchcraft, the underworld, and the spirits that reside there. It can be used in shamanic journeying and opening gateways to the otherworld. It has applications in dark magic for overcoming the will and causing forgetfulness. The thorn-covered pods may be used in protective charms and hexes. (Thorn apple, aka datura, is discussed further in chapter 6.)

White horehound (*Marrubium vulgare*): This plant protects one from magic and also delivers clarity to the mind during ritual. It can be used to strengthen mental powers. Due to its medicinal properties it can be used to expel spiritual parasites. Both white horehound and black horehound belong to the Lamiaceae family, which is a large group of plants known as mint or deadnettle.

PLANTS OF HEALING AND MAGIC

Aztec Tobacco (*Nicotiana rustica*): Cleansing and Conjuration

A member of the nightshade family, *Nicotiana rustica* is known as Aztec tobacco, wild tobacco, and strong tobacco. Tobacco, like cannabis, has been cultivated by humans for such a long time that there is no longer an original strain, and we cannot be sure of its true origins. The genus *Nicotiana* is generally assumed to have originated in the New

World, though that claim has been disputed by some. Seeds have been discovered in Egyptian tombs, suggesting the possibility of contact via trade between the Egyptians and Mesoamericans. *N. rustica* is no longer grown in the United States, having been replaced by other varieties like *N. tabacum.*

N. rustica contains harmala alkaloids in addition to its nicotine content. These are the same alkaloids that give Syrian rue its entheogenic properties. The nicotine content of tobacco plants varies widely. *N. rustica* is more potent and can have a nicotine content of up to 18 percent. *N. tabacum* has a nicotine content of 0.5 to 9 percent and at its strongest is only half as potent as *N. rustica* (Furbee 2009). The leaves have the highest nicotine content, followed by the stems and root. The flowers also contain small amounts of nicotine and can be included in smoking blends and ritual incense.

Tobacco is used by many cultures in shamanic ritual and for its entheogenic properties. It has a long history of use in the shamanic traditions of the Americas and is used extensively by shamans to travel to other realities and communicate with entities in other realms. Tobacco has qualities that make it stimulating, relaxing, and narcotic. It has also been used as an emetic, diuretic, and antiseptic. It also has been employed as a natural insecticide and vermicide and can be made into infusions to keep pests out of gardens.

Tobacco has many ritual applications, and it is sacred to Native Americans and South American shamans and has been adopted by African diasporic traditions. It is a plant of conjuration, given as food for spirits in the form of smoke. It is used in cleansing and healing rituals as a spiritual restorative that is blown over the body. The sacred smoke was used against spirits of disease to cure the sick. Cigarettes and cigars make common offerings, and the smoke is often blown over an altar or images of deities and other spirits. The juice of the leaves can be pressed and reserved for shamanic purposes.

Powdered wild tobacco is used as a ritual snuff known as *rapé.* Snuff was also popular in Europe for a time. Tobacco was first introduced to England by Sir Walter Raleigh in 1586 and met violent oppression by the monarchy and papacy. In other parts of Europe, it was known as *Hyoscyamus peruvianus* or Peruvian henbane until 1650.

Hunting parties would use the plant to cleanse their head and give them focus when out on excursions. The Caruña people would drip the juice into their eyes in order to enhance night vision and to see spirits and discern between good and evil. The tobacco spirit was sought out as an intermediary to bring about contact with other entities. The juice mixed with lime (calcium hydroxide) is applied to the inside of elbows, wrists, or back of the head. The alkalinity of the lime makes absorption of the alkaloids more effective.

Tobacco is a food for the gods and the spirits, which may explain the addictive effects it has on humankind. It is a sacrament that has been turned into a commodity, and the spirit of tobacco has repaid its exploitation with addiction and health problems. When approached with reverence and respect in ceremony, it is a powerful ally still willing to work with those who treat it as the sacrament it was intended to be.

※

Clary Sage (*Salvia sclarea*): Clarity and Clairvoyance

Salvia sclarea belongs to the *Salvia* genus, the largest in the mint family. It is related to diviner's sage, *Salvia divinorum*. Clary comes from the Latin *claris,* meaning "clear," because of its use in eye treatments. Clary sage is used in ayurvedic medicine to balance the three *doshas*, representing the energy of the five elements within an individual. It is considered the most euphoric of the essential oils, producing an almost narcotic effect. It has pronounced antidepressant qualities and is a powerful aid to easing depression, anxiety, and stress. It is both intoxicating, sensuous, and uplifting (Farrer-Halls 2005). The effects of clary sage are warming and sedative. It is used as a nerve tonic, producing mild euphoria and a sense of well-being. Dreaming is enhanced by using the essential oil before sleep.

Clary sage can also be used to treat sexual dysfunction, impotency, and frigidity by its aphrodisiac properties. It can be made into a massage oil. It contains a chemical known as sclerol, an estrogen-like structure with hormone-balancing effects. It can help with menstrual pain and perimenopause symptoms. It has a stimulating effect on the uterus and should be avoided by pregnant women until the end of the third trimester. For pain relief, clary sage can be added to a hot bath to relax tension and soothe pain.

Magically, clary sage can be used in ritual to travel to the underworld. It may be used in liminal rites for its ability to balance light and darkness. It is a lunar herb and is associated with glamour magic and deception through disguise. Alternatively, it allows the user to see through the pretenses of others. As a dreaming herb, it enhances vividness and recall, making it an effective herb for prophetic dreaming. When used ritually, it can be combined with other essential oils to aid in meditation and trance.

✥

Hazel (*Corylus avellana*): Tree of Wisdom

The hazel tree is ruled by the planet Mercury. In Celtic mythology, the hazelnut is the source of food and knowledge for the Salmon of Wisdom. In Scandinavian mythology, the hazel was consecrated to the god Thor. It was mentioned in the poetic Edda to be a symbol of sovereignty and was used to make scepters for kings (Folkard 1884, 190). Hazel wood is the traditional wood of the magician's wand. A forked hazel branch, called Moses's rod, is used in dowsing to find buried treasure, and the caduceus of Hermes was made of a hazel branch.

The caduceus, a symbol of the medical profession, is a hazel rod with wings around which are coiled two serpents. The connection between serpents and hazel continues. Snakes are associated with Mercury and are symbols of wisdom, healing, and transformation. They are also symbols of occult mystery and knowledge. In Roman mythology, land spirits or genii loci were depicted as giant snakes beneath the earth. The witch and the *wurm* are brethren under the horned one. The mythical *Huzelwurm* of Germanic lore dwells in the roots of the hazel tree, imparting wisdom to those able to discern its presence. This creature was said to be a white horned snake that lived in the roots of the tree, and if you were able to catch it and eat it, you would gain knowledge of the occult forces. Hazelnuts were used to protect against snake bites, and the wood was used to cure them.

Myrrh (*Commiphora myrrha*): Fragrant Euphoriant

Myrrh resin was an important commodity in the ancient world. It was used by the ancient Egyptians in their embalming process because of its powerful preservative capabilities. The resin extracted from this small, thorny shrub has been used throughout history as a ritual fumigant. Myrrh is thought to be the lunar counterpart to frankincense, which is solar in nature. Myrrh can be used in incense for lunar workings, divination, spirit work, and necromancy. There are many different varieties of myrrh, which vary in quality and scent. It has a sweet, earthy scent, which pairs well with many other herbs as an incense. It is particularly suited for burning during meditation and trance work.

Since ancient times, the entheogenic effects of myrrh have been known. It was included in an incense recipe used by Levite priests, mentioned in the Torah, which contained galbanum, two types of myrrh, saffron, agarwood, cinnamon, and cassia (Leviticus 16:12), all of which are known for their effects, including their role as opiate receptor agonists. They activate the opiate receptors in a way that is similar to actual opiates, resulting in euphoria, a stimulated sense of relaxation, and a sense of warm fuzziness. Myrrh along with frankincense is classed as a tranquilizer due to its effects on GABA receptors.

Myrrh, along with cinnamon and cassia, contains essential oil derivatives known as allylbenzenes. These chemicals are known for their medicinal action and documented psychoactivity. They are closely related to psychoactive alkaloids and stimulants. These chemicals have a mild effect on human physiology unless coupled with the appropriate enzyme inhibitors. Inhibitors like nutmeg are used in synergy with allylbenzene-containing plants to produce more pronounced effects, a reaction that was known to the ancient Egyptians, who used these ingredients in a massage oil that was reserved for the pharaoh. The physical effects of the massage, which dilated the surface capillaries, along with these synergistic plants resulted in an enhanced effect.

The effects of myrrh terpene isolates or myrrh extract have been likened to the effects of kratom, a tropical evergreen tree whose leaves, when dried, powdered, and eaten, produce an opiate-like effect. Myrrh resin has traditionally been chewed in small amounts, smoked, or infused into wine and drunk. The dark-red tincture of myrrh also yields an extract that can be smoked, taken sublingually, or insufflated. The tincture is macerated for two to four weeks and then separated from the remaining marc. The extract is poured onto a glass baking dish and the solvent evaporated so that the remaining extract can be scraped off with a razor. It is this extract that is taken, in dosages of 50 to 100 mg, for its entheogenic properties or added to ritual incense or smoking blends.

Snowdrop (*Galanthus nivalis*): Protector and Antidote

In Homer's *Odyssey*, the sorceress Circe, who is knowledgeable of poisons, gives Odysseus's men "food mixed with evil drugs," a magical potion that turns them into swine. Some have suggested that the poison given to Odysseus's men was some type of hallucinogenic nightshade. The god Hermes comes to Odysseus's aid and gives him a strange plant to protect him from Circe's enchantments. This plant is described as "black at the root with a flower as white as milk." He calls the plant *moly* but does not provide a definitive description of what it is. Many have theorized as to the identity of moly, but there is no clear evidence of its identity.

One of the most convincing arguments for the identity of moly was put forth by Andreas Plaitakis and Roger Duvoisin, who pointed to snowdrop as the mythical plant (Plaitakis and Duvoisin 1983). The chemical action of snowdrop as an anticholinesterase is particularly interesting. An anticholinesterase is an acetylcholinesterase inhibitor, meaning that it inhibits the breakdown of acetylcholine, increasing its level and duration. The tropane alkaloids block acetylcholine at nerve receptors due to their anticholinergic effects. An anticholinesterase would reverse the central actions of a tropane alkaloid. One of the chemicals in the bulb of the snowdrop, galanthamine, is just such an anticholinesterase. The description of the effects of moly by Homer suggest such a chemical action. In such a case, this would be the first example of an anticholinesterase drug being used to prevent or reverse poisoning by tropane alkaloids (Plaitakis and Duvoisin 1983). (For a list of other antidotes for alkaloids, see the box at the end of chapter 9.)

Snowdrop flowers in early February and is associated with Candlemas. It was introduced to Great Britain by monks. It is a symbol of purity but also of death because it resembles a shrouded corpse. It was used occasionally in ancient Greece for neuralgia and pain.

※

Syrian Rue (*Peganum harmala*): The Bitterest Herb

Syrian rue grows in the eastern Mediterranean, the Middle East, and parts of Asia including the Indian peninsula. Harmel is one of many names associated with this legendary plant, known in the ancient world as moly, as listed by Dioscorides. However, there is no irrefutable evidence of an association of this plant with the moly given to Odysseus by Hermes in the *Odyssey* to break Circe's enchantment. Such an association is evidence of Syrian rue's prominence in the ancient world. It had an extensive reputation as an apotropaic and would have been known as such by Homer.

In Africa, the Mediterranean, and the Middle East, it has been used to treat mental illness, as an abortifacient, and as a talisman against the evil eye. It was sometimes used as an aphrodisiac and for its mood-elevating effects. Magically, it is considered a Saturnian herb and is used as a ritual entheogen and in protection magic. Syrian rue is traditionally burned to ward off evil spirits and to prevent misfortune. Avicenna (980–1037 CE), a Persian physician, mentions its use as a visionary plant and by the Sufis to enhance their trances.

The seeds of Syrian rue are used for their entheogenic effects; they are smoked or burned and inhaled for psychotropic effects. They have a sedative and narcotic effect similar to opium, with mild to moderate visual hallucinations. The seeds can be chewed to absorb their compounds orally; however, they are incredibly bitter and unpalatable. Infusions and tinctures using lemon juice or alcohol have been employed. It is said that infusing the seeds in hot water produces less nausea than other methods. Small doses of the seeds (25 to 50 mg) have a mild stimulating effect and can cause agitation or act as a depressant. Taking 2.5 g of the seeds whole will result in a slight loss of coordination, but some sources say that as little as 1 g of seeds can cause hallucinations. Larger doses (300 to 750 mg) have a hallucinogenic effect (Yuruktumen 2008). Higher doses of 3 to 5 g of the seeds, powdered and placed in gel caps, are taken for their psychotropic effects.

Syrian rue contains the chemicals harmine and harmaline. Harmaline solutions, like other alkaloid-containing extracts, are fluorescent under a black light. Harmaline alkaloids are MAOIs and should not be taken in conjunction with MAOI medicines.

Caution: As Syrian rue is an abortifacient, pregnant women should not take it.

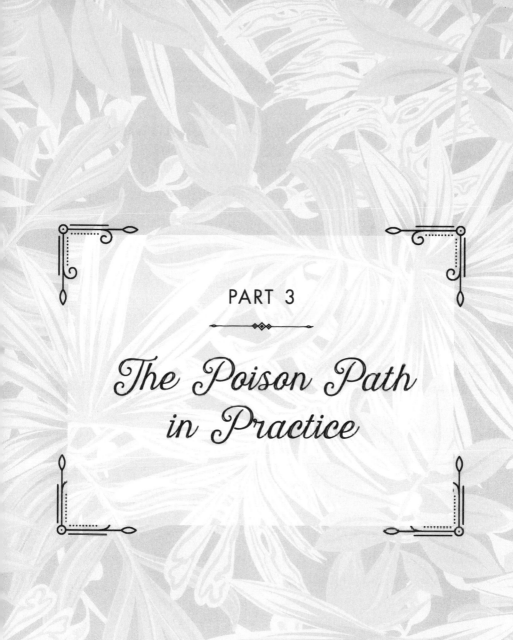

PART 3

The Poison Path
in Practice

9

Walking the Crooked Path
Preparation and Formulation

*T*his chapter focuses on the preparation of both baneful and more benign plants for their use in medicine and in formulas designed for ritual. Some of the plants we have discussed in previous chapters are too dangerous for any kind of ingestion, even topical application. Plants like wolfsbane, foxglove, and hemlock should never be ingested, and applying them to the skin is also risky, at best causing skin irritation. Alkaloids are absorbed through the skin, and while topical application is much safer than ingesting, it is not without its risks.

Many of the entheogens mentioned in this book, such as mugwort, wormwood, and myrrh, are safe to use as long as basic herbal preparation guidelines are followed. There are many resources available that give instructions for making your own herbal medicines, including tinctures, salves, and fluid extracts. In this chapter, I focus on the preparation of ritual oils, ointments, and other recipes, all of which may be used both medicinally and ritually.

Nightshades are anti-inflammatory and antispasmodic and are effective for relieving pain, such as sciatica nerve pain and all types of muscle pain. They are a great substitute for addictive painkillers and can be used in synergy with other soothing plants. They have a calming and sedating effect in most individuals, but in some people, they can be more stimulating and euphoric.

Ritually, these plants serve many purposes and are indispensable tools that enhance one's practice. Through their ability to relax the mind and open our perception to subtle realities, they are great for any kind of trance work. Nightshades have been used by many ancient cultures for prophesying and as an aid to divination. They make reaching altered states of consciousness much easier. In addition to honing in our perception on spiritual energies, the nightshades are also used to attract spirits. Many of them have been used by traditional people for centuries as offerings to spirits, gods, and the dead.

EXTRACTION METHODS

Many of the formulas in this book incorporate plants from the nightshade family, which contain tropane alkaloids. Alkaloids are soluble in both organic solvents (alcohol) and fats (vegetable oils and animal fat). Tropane alkaloids can be extracted from Solanaceae plants using all the usual means, such as a water or oil infusion or alcohol extraction. Acids such as vinegar and red wine can also be used. Acids convert alkaloids to their salt form, which makes them easier to absorb. Tropane alkaloids are water soluble, which means that they extract more readily in solutions containing water. This also means that they do not extract as easily into oil. Many of the formulas that we will be using are oil based. There are a few techniques that can compensate for this issue. Depending on the desired use and necessary mode of delivery, alcohol tinctures, infused oils, and ointments are all potential options. In some cases, a water infusion or decoction can be made for topical use, but these plants are not recommended to be brewed into a tea and drunk. Ingesting alkaloids in this way is risky and leads to rather unpleasant experiences.

Tropane alkaloids are readily absorbed through the skin and mucous membranes. Tinctures, oils, and ointments are all effective means of delivery for topical use. The only nightshades that are safe for use on or near mucous membranes are mandrake and henbane. Some nightshades like belladonna and datura cause irritation in some individuals when applied to the skin. Applying formulas on or near mucous membranes—the thin capillary-dense tissues near entrances to the body—causes the alkaloids to go straight to the bloodstream, which has a potential for overdose and other overwhelming experiences. Here are some basic terms to know when researching these preparations.

Maceration: This is the process of submerging plant material in a solvent to extract the active components.

Menstruum: This is a term for the solvent, the liquid in which the herb is submerged. Water, vinegar, alcohol, and oil can all be used as potential menstruums or solvents.

Marc: The plant material, also known as the *solute*. This is the material that is submerged in the solvent or menstruum.

Comminution: The reduction of herbal material to an optimum particle size. This increases the surface area of the material and helps break down the cell walls of the plant, making the process more efficient. Fresh plant material can be finely chopped or placed in a freezer to break down cell walls. Dry plant material can be pulverized using a mortar and pestle or coffee grinder. Powdered plant material in a solvent must be shaken every day to compensate for settling at the bottom, which can impede the extraction process.

Aerial parts: These are the parts of the plant that grow above the ground. Flowers and leaves take up more space in a container and should be finely cut; otherwise, an excessive amount of menstruum is needed, resulting in a more diluted product.

Dense materials: The roots and bark constitute the dense materials. The denser the material, the longer the extraction process. Hard roots, bark, and resin should be reduced in size for more efficient maceration.

Weight-to-volume ratio: This tells you how much plant material is used (weight) in relation to the amount of menstruum (volume). For healing herbs known as balms, the optimum ratio for the most concentrated product is just enough menstruum to cover the plant material. In the folk tincture method, the menstruum should be at least one inch above the surface of the plant material to avoid oxidation. When the plant material is finely comminuted, less menstruum is needed. The less menstruum used, the more concentrated the product. The weight-to-volume ratio for nonbaneful herbs or balms is higher. The ratio of 1 part plant material to 5 parts menstruum is the higher limit. Usually a ratio of 1:4 or 1:3 is used for leafier herbs, while 1:2 or 1:1 is used for denser material, such as roots and seeds.

Weights and Measurements

Alcohol at 190 proof (95 percent) is used diluted with water. High-proof alcohol is unstable and should not be taken unless diluted. The percentage ratios of water to alcohol are as follows:

1 part water to 2 parts alcohol = 60 percent

1 part water to 1 part alcohol = 45 percent

2 parts water to 1 part alcohol = 30 percent

3 parts water to 1 part alcohol = 25 percent

ABBREVIATIONS

fluid ounce: floz (apothecary) or fl. oz. (modern)

fluidram or fluidrachm: fldr

gallon: gal.

gram: g

milligram: mg

milliliter: ml

minim: min

ounce: oz.

pint: pt.

quart: qt.

tablespoon: Tbsp.

teaspoon: tsp.

Apothecary System of Measurement

VOLUME

min (smallest unit) = 1 drop

60 min = 1 fldr

1 fldr = 1 tsp. or 5 ml

1 grain = 60 mg

4 fldr = ½ floz = 1 Tbsp. or 15 ml

8 fldr = 1 floz = 2 Tbsp. or 30 ml

16 floz = 1 pt.

2 pt. = 32 floz = 1 qt.

Modern Measurements

VOLUME

½ cup = 4 fl. oz. = 125 ml

2 cups = 16 fl. oz. = 500 ml

DRY MEASURE EQUIVALENTS

3 tsp. = 1 Tbsp. = ½ oz.

2 Tbsp. = ⅛ cup = 1 oz. = 28.3 g

INFUSED OILS

Oils are one way of working with baneful herbs. They are easy to make and are a little safer than using alcohol extraction. Oils extract a smaller amount of the alkaloids than alcohol, resulting in a less concentrated product.

Infused oils can be made using heat, or the plant material can be allowed to infuse naturally. Heating the oil containing the dry plant material is faster than letting it macerate naturally and is more effective at extracting the alkaloids which is desirable for entheogenic formulations. The infusion is the same quality; it is just less green in color. If you use a double boiler or slow cooker, heat the infusion on a low temperature for four to six hours. When macerating naturally, the dried plant material is added to the oil in a glass jar and sealed. Keep the jar in a warm place, out of direct sunlight, for four to six weeks or longer and shake regularly. Many practitioners use the lunar cycle to determine this process, either starting on the new moon or using a specific astrological aspect.

To create a more concentrated and effective oil, the herbs can first be extracted into alcohol. This is called the alcohol-intermediary method and is used in medicinal herbalism to create stronger infused oils. Alkaloids are water soluble and infuse into alcohol more readily than oil. A small amount of vodka (approximately one shot glass per ounce) can be poured over the dry plant material. This initiates the extraction process, making it more effective. This concentrated tincture can then be added to the oil. The oil and alcohol are then boiled together until the alcohol boils off and there is no separation. This technique should be done outdoors or in a well-ventilated area.

Dry plant material is commonly used to make oils because the water content in fresh plant material can contribute to spoilage in an oil; however, fresh plant material can be cooked in oil, something that was done in the past. Fresh plant material is placed directly into the oil in a pan and cooked on medium-high heat, being careful not to overcook it. The water content in the fresh plant material is evaporated as the oil is heated, leaving behind the active components. It is important to ensure all of the water has evaporated after the plant material has been strained out. If there are any remaining water droplets, continue to heat the oil. This will ensure that the oil doesn't spoil.

Oils can be used topically or for anointing ritual objects. They can also be thickened with beeswax to create ointments. Essential oils may be added for their influence or for preservation. Rosemary essential oil, benzoin resinoid, or poplar buds can be added to the infusion for their antimicrobial properties. Vitamin E oil is commonly added as a natural preservative.

TINCTURES

Tinctures or alcohol extracts are easy to make, require little material, and last indefinitely. Tinctures are concentrated medicinal products that are typically taken orally by putting a few drops into a glass of water. They can also be used to infuse concentrated herbal components into oils and ointments. Medicinal tinctures using more potent baneful herbs are typically made with dried plant material at a much lower ratio, creating a safer and more diluted product. Fresh plant material can also be tinctured, keeping in mind that it contains more alkaloids than dry. Using a higher ratio of alcohol and plant material will compensate for the increased concentration in fresh plant material. The water content of the plants will slightly lower the percentage of alcohol. Medicinal weight-to-volume ratios for nightshades are usually 1:10, and these tinctures are used homeopathically. A higher ratio of 1:4 or 1:5 can be used as a general guideline when creating more concentrated products for entheogenic use. This is a general guideline and the ratio can be adjusted for individual needs and the varying concentration of alkaloids in the plant material.

Tinctures are made using alcohol as the menstruum; either ethyl alcohol or ethanol (drinking alcohol) is used. Rubbing alcohol should not be used to make tinctures or ingested. Typically, a grain alcohol such as vodka or Everclear is used, but some traditional recipes will use other alcohols such as brandy. Tinctures can be made using dry or fresh plant material. When using fresh plant material, the water content must be taken into consideration since it will dilute the alcohol slightly.

Alcohol breaks down plant cells and destroys enzymes. Many of the herbal constituents that are poorly soluble in water will break down in alcohol. Glycosides and other constituents are more stable in alcohol than in other solvents. Medicinal tinctures use a dilution of alcohol in water, with 25 percent being the standard. Some herbs require higher percentages of alcohol to water.

Recipes for tinctures are written with the ratio of plant material to solvent and the percentage of solvent and water. For example, 1:2, 60 percent means twice as much solvent as plant material with the solvent composed of one part water and two parts alcohol. A percentage of 25 percent would be three parts water (75 percent) to one part alcohol.

Once the herbs and menstruum are combined, the tincture is left to macerate for a period; the timing varies from a couple of weeks to an entire moon cycle or a couple of months. The tincture must be shaken regularly during this period. Daniel Schulke, in his book *Ars Philtron*, suggests beginning a tincture on the new moon and allowing it to macerate for one lunation. This follows the moon's gestation period; as the moon grows, so does the energy within the tincture. Once the process is complete, the spent marc is strained out. It can be added to a new menstruum to create a dilute tincture that can be used for future maceration to create a more concentrated product.

Fresh Tinctures

Due to the water content of fresh plants, fresh tinctures are slightly diluted. In the case of herbs containing alkaloids, the fresher the material, the higher the alkaloid content. This goes for dried plant material as well. Baneful herbs that have been recently dried have a higher alkaloid content than those that have been stored for a year, since the alkaloids degrade over time. A slightly diluted tincture is not a major concern when working with these potent plants. There are some benefits to working with fresh plant material. In *Ars Philtron,* Schulke comments on the use of fresh herbal material, pointing out some of the benefits and differences.

Schulke infers that spagyric alchemists prefer dry plant material, while folk magicians prefer fresh. He states that the governing genus or spirit of the plant is more alive and connected to its parental plant in fresh herbage. This makes fresh herbs more effective for idols and homunculi, using the tincture as a living potion to connect with the plant spirit familiar, or as a means of preserving the physical body of the plant in its own tincture as a spirit vessel. He also notes that fresh herbs, due to their water content, contain a more Mercurian aspect, while dry herbs contain more salt and sulfur. This will come into play when making spagyric tinctures, which contain all three alchemical components. He suggests pulverizing half of the fresh plant material while leaving the other half whole because of natural preservative enzymes that exist within the cell wall.

Fresh tinctures are made in the same way as tinctures of dried plants with higher weight-to-volume ratios to compensate for the fresh plants' water content. The resulting tincture is more energetic and more therapeutic.

Spagyric Tinctures

Making spagyric tinctures is one of the main practices of the plant alchemist. The making of the tincture is a ritualized and powerful experience and can be enhanced through astrological timing. These tinctures are more energetically whole, containing the entirety of the plant matter. Their effects are more powerful and more medicinally beneficial.

In alchemical extraction, plant parts are first altered and then recombined, a process that recognizes the importance of the synergy of the whole plant (DeKorne 1994). By dissolving and recombining, the creator follows the alchemical process of *solve et coagula,* creating a powerful bond with the resulting product. This is a powerful way to begin working with these plants as spirit familiars. The living tincture can be used to empower other formulas and can be kept on the altar as a means of contacting the plant spirit familiar. Once the tincture is complete, a homunculus can be created by adding the roots, leaves, stems, flowers, and seeds of one or more plant spirit familiars to be preserved in the tincture. Folk tinctures are also made using the entire plant.

In spagyric tincture making, the plant material is powdered and mixed with water until it makes a pourable paste. This is spread out on a baking sheet lined with plastic wrap and the water is allowed to evaporate. The alchemist then grinds the remains into a fine powder. The powder is added to menstruum and allowed to macerate for a predetermined period of time; the tincture is shaken regularly. After this initial period, the spent marc is filtered and pressed. It is spread out on a baking sheet again to be calcinated. The process of calcination uses heat to reduce the plant material to its alchemical salt. The alcohol-containing marc can be lit on fire and burned to ash. The ash is then placed in an oven until it is reduced to a gray-white ash. This can take anywhere from six to ten hours; the ashes should occasionally be stirred and redistributed. It is important to keep the layer of ashes thin to maximize the surface area.

The ash, which is the alchemical salt, is recombined with the tincture and allowed to macerate for another one to two weeks, shaken daily. The new spagyric tincture is then filtered again, the filtrate is discarded, and the tincture is finished. This creates an energetically whole entity. It opens the plant, creating stronger curative properties. When made with plants that are not toxic, the tincture can be evaporated, and the remaining dry residue can be collected and ingested or added to other formulas. This is not recommended for baneful herbs because the resulting residue is too concentrated. The spagyric tincture can be used ritually and incorporated into formulas that are not meant for ingestion. The process of preparing the spagyric tincture can bring new insight into the energetic nature of these plants and their spirits.

When working with plants that contain alkaloids, pH is taken into consideration and can be used to create a more potent and holistic formula. While alkaloids are readily extracted by alcohol, vinegar can be used because of its acidic pH, creating a vinegar tincture. The alkaloids are converted to their salts by acidic solutions, making them more available to the human body. For this process, pure apple cider vinegar should be used.

A mixture that is 55 percent undiluted alcohol, 35 percent water, and 10 percent vinegar is used as the menstruum. For example, if you wanted to make 100 ml of tincture you would combine 55 ml of high-proof alcohol, 35 ml water, and 10 ml apple cider vinegar.

FLUID EXTRACTS

Fluid extracts are alcoholic extracts prepared using a 1:1 weight-to-volume ratio, resulting in a concentrated tincture. Traditionally, tinctures are prepared by maceration, while fluid extracts are prepared by cold percolation. By creating a fluid extract in this way, using a 1:1 ratio, you are creating an extract that is the equivalent to taking 1 g dried herb per 1 ml of extract. For milder herbs, this provides a more convenient dose range in a more condensed product, rather than having to take larger amounts of a more diluted tincture. When using chemically potent plants like belladonna, the dosage is very small. Typically, fluid extracts of this kind would be diluted or infused into oil for the creation of ointments.

Many herbal remedies use the volatile oils of plants that are easily extracted into alcohol. Plant alkaloids are readily extracted through this process. However, some plants and fungi contain complex polysaccharides that extract only through boiling. A tincture can be made using *Amanita muscaria,* for example; afterward, the marc is pressed and decocted in boiling water and allowed to evaporate to a low volume. The spent marc is added to a pan and barely covered with water. It is boiled vigorously for two to four hours, with water added as needed. The marc is filtered, and the alcoholic tincture is added to the remaining fluid and simmered gently until the mixture becomes thick and no longer separates. This decoction contains all the extracted components of the marc, along with the tincture.

Great care must be taken when creating fluid extracts from baneful herbs because of their increased concentration. Liquid-liquid extraction is an advanced process that involves adding the fluid extract to the proper amount of oil and boiling to evaporate the alcohol. Through this process, the alkaloids extracted by the alcohol are infused into the oil, and larger quantities can be made without having to use large amounts of plant material.

DETERMINING ALKALOID CONTENT FOR DOSAGES

It is important to remember that the alkaloid content of tropane-alkaloid-containing plants varies widely. It is based on a number of factors, such as the freshness of the plant material, the time of year it was harvested, and the growing conditions. Scientific measurements also vary from one source to another and only provide an approximate range. The actual alkaloid content of an individual plant can be much lower or much higher.

For example, *Atropa belladonna* has an overall alkaloid content of 0.28 to 0.32 percent. To determine the alkaloid content of one gram of plant material in milligrams, multiply the percentage by 1,000 (the number of milligrams per gram).

1 g = 1,000 mg × 0.28%–0.32% = 2.8–3.2 mg per 1 g of plant material

28 gr (1 oz.) = 28,000 mg × 0.3% or 0.003 = 84 mg per oz.

An average single dose of 0.5–1 g of plant material contains 0.15–3 mg of alkaloids.

MEDICINAL NIGHTSHADE RECIPES

Most of the following recipes are from a 1934 book called *The Herbalist,* written by Joseph E. Meyer, an herbalist, publisher, illustrator, and supplier of pharmaceutical-grade herbs. Many of his herbs were grown at the Indiana Botanic Gardens, a retail store founded in 1910; his love for plants allowed him to grow this large multimillion-dollar business. He wrote extensively on the medicinal and folkloric uses of herbs by different cultures.

While the tea recipes included here are presented in their entirety, they are not exhaustive in their information. These are examples of actual medical prescriptions that were used into the twentieth century. Where the tincture ratios are missing, it is safe to assume that Meyer intended a 1:10 or 1:20 ratio, which is commonly used in these types of preparations, though we cannot say for certain. These examples also give us insight into our own preparations and experimentations as we explore these botanicals. This is important because it shows that these herbs are not so poisonous that they are beyond working with, and their use is not confined to the Middle Ages or earlier.

ᘓᕦᕤ

Bittersweet Nightshade Tea for Skin Irritations
(Meyer 1934, 17)

- ✿ 2 tsp. *Solanum dulcamara* root
- ✿ 1 pt. boiling water

Steep root in boiling water. Drink cold two to three teaspoons, six times per day. Tincture dosage: 10–20 drops.

ᘓᕦᕤ

Belladonna Tea
(Meyer 1934, 13–14)

- ✿ 1 tsp. *Atropa belladonna* leaves
- ✿ 1 pt. boiling water

Steep leaves in boiling water. Drink one to two teaspoons cold, two to three times per day. This tea has energetic, narcotic, anodyne, antispasmodic, calmative, and relaxant properties. Tincture dosage: ½–1 drop.

ᘓᕦᕤ

Black Nightshade Tea
(Meyer 1934, 48)

- ✿ 1–2 tsp. *Solanum nigrum* leaves
- ✿ 1 qt. boiling water

Steep leaves in boiling water. Take liquid one teaspoon at a time. Tincture dosage: ½–1 drop. This tea is somewhat narcotic and sedative.

Meyer notes that in large doses, *Solanum nigrum* causes sickness and vertigo and copious perspiration and purging the next day. He also mentions its use as an ointment.

❧❧

Carolina Horsenettle Tea
(Meyer 1934)

*Horsenettle is an interesting member of the nightshade family that
grows across the eastern and southern parts of North America.
It has white to light purple star-shaped flowers with a large yellow
stamen similar to bittersweet nightshade but larger.*

- 1 tsp. *Solanum carolinense* root
- 1 cup boiling water

Steep root in boiling water for one-half hour. Take one-half cupful at
night or one mouthful three times per day; one to two cups may be
taken. Tincture dosage: ½–1 fldr.

Meyer further notes that a poultice of *Solanum carolinense* leaves
may be used to treat poison ivy rashes. The berries and root are anodyne, aphrodisiac, and diuretic and have been used to treat epilepsy. An
infusion of the seeds can be gargled for a sore throat.

❧❧

Henbane-Infused Honey

*Honey is an amazing preservative and can last indefinitely when
stored in the right conditions. Archaeologists have found pots of honey
in ancient Egyptian tombs that are around three thousand years old
and still edible. Honey can be infused with virtually any herb, and
the process is as simple as making a tincture or an infused oil.*

- 2 oz. henbane, dried and chopped
- Raw honey (preferably local)

Add the plant material to a one-quart glass jar and cover with honey.
Use the back of a wooden spoon to ensure all the honey makes it to the
bottom of the jar. Seal the jar and keep in a warm area like a window-
sill. The warmth from the sunlight will help the infusion process. The
longer the herbs infuse in the honey, the stronger it will be. Infuse for
two to four weeks, turning the jar upside down at least once a day. Once

complete, strain out the herbs and store the honey in a cool dark place.

Add one to three teaspoons of honey to tea made from bitter herbs such as mugwort. The honey can also be eaten by itself, used in other recipes, or spread on biscuits.

THE CHUMASH AND SACRED DATURA

The Chumash, a Native American tribe, historically inhabited the central and southern coastal regions of California and still live in the area today. The Chumash people used *Datura wrightii* or sacred datura, known as *momoy* in the Chumash language, for medicinal and spiritual purposes. Momoy was also the name of the spirit of the plant. Momoy was a wise grandmother who retained the lore of the sacred datura. The Chumash people would chew on a small part of the leaf to protect their spirits. Momoy was used in topical preparations to relieve moderate to severe pain. The topical preparation is safe and effective, delivering small amounts of active ingredients locally. It disrupts the pain cycle through the sensory nerves and prevents systemic toxicity (Adams and Wang 2015). The leaves and flowers were combined with tobacco to make a strong bath for acute arthritic pain, injuries, and overworked muscles. The person would soak in the bath until he or she began feeling relaxed, not staying in for too long.

The sacred datura was also used for its visionary properties. Chumash myth says that drinking the water that Momoy washed her hands in (datura infusion) would bring visions of the future and spiritual guides. Drinking too much of the infusion would lead to a terrible fate. There were many guidelines and taboos surrounding the use of the plant. If the guidelines were not followed and the plant was not treated with respect, the plant spirit would become hostile. Some of the prescribed guidelines were not indulging in meat, greasy foods, or sex before using the plant. Tobacco, however, could be smoked since it was believed that Momoy consumed tobacco for sustenance.

The Chumash people also made an infusion of momoy as a foot bath for pain. They made a sun tea of seven leaves and seven flowers from the *D. wrightii* plant. The medicine is absorbed through the pores in the feet to reach the specific area needing relief. It also helps with abrasions and bruises, arthritis pain, overexertion, back and neck pain, and joint pain and works as an overall restorative, relaxing the entire body (Adams and Wang 2015).

❧

Momoy Foot Soak
(Adams and Garcia 2005)

- 0.25 kg *Datura wrightii* roots and/or stems
- 1 liter water

Infuse the mixture in the sun for three days. When ready, strain the fluid and heat to slightly warmer than body temperature. The feet are soaked for fifteen to twenty minutes. Some people may need to soak their feet every night to become more relaxed and receptive to spirit.

OINTMENTS AND INCENSE

❧

Unguentum Populeon
(Green 2010, 130)

Poplar ointments have been used in medicine for centuries. This early recipe comes from the Trotula, *a twelfth-century medical text, and is for those who are unable to sleep. The unguent is rubbed on the temples and other pulse points and on the palms of the hands and soles of the feet.*

- 1½ pounds poplar buds (*Oculus populi*)
- 2 pounds unsalted pork fat
- 3 oz. each: red poppy, mandrake leaves, fresh tips of bramble, henbane, black nightshade, common stonecrop, wild lettuce, house leek, burdock, violet, pennywort
- 5 liters high-quality wine

First pound the poplar buds separately and then again with the fat. Let the fat and bud mixture sit for two days. On the third day, gather all the herbs and, separately, grind each one thoroughly. Mix the ground herbs with the fat mixture and form into little lozenges. Put the lozenges in a pan and add enough wine to cover the lozenges. Boil the wine until it evaporates, stirring constantly; the fat will dissolve into the wine. After straining the mixture through cheesecloth, set the strained mixture aside to cool. Store in a vase.

Unguentum Populeum

This recipe was included in The Dispensatory of the United States of America *(Remington 1918) and attributed to the French Codex.*

- 100 g dried white poppy leaves
- 100 g dried belladonna leaves
- 100 g dried henbane leaves
- 100 g dried black nightshade leaves
- 400 g alcohol
- 4,000 g lard
- 800 g poplar buds

Moisten the leaves with the alcohol and allow them to macerate in a closed container for twenty-four hours. Add lard to the mixture and heat gently for three hours, stirring frequently. Add crushed poplar buds and allow to infuse for ten hours over gentle heat. The resulting ointment is strained and cooled. This ointment was used throughout Europe as an anodyne, applied to painful areas.

Incense for Meditative Trance and Divination
(Rätsch 2005, 82)

Ritual fumigations are a common means for the evocation of spirits.
The smoke provides them with energy and a medium in which to
manifest. Burned offerings have been used to feed spirits for centuries.
It was believed that deities and spirits gained sustenance from
pleasing aromas and that burning the offering multiplied its power.

- 1 part belladonna leaves and flowers
- 1 part fool's parsley
- 1 part acorns
- 1 part vervain
- 1 part peppermint
- 1 part thistle

To make the incense, combine the ingredients in an earthenware bowl.

Incense for the Dead

This incense blend is specifically formulated for working with the spirits of the dead, including ancestral spirits, ghosts, and the spirits that preside over them. It can be burned as an offering or in rituals to summon spirits. Not only does it give the spirits a means to materialize, it also enhances the magician's ability to see them.

- 1 Tbsp. each: dittany of Crete, skullcap, mugwort, wild lettuce, mullein
- 1 pinch each: henbane seeds, tobacco, cardamom pods

To make the incense, combine the ingredients in an earthenware bowl. The blend can be jarred and interred in the ground from new moon to new moon to imbue the blend with additional chthonic energy.

RECIPES FOR MAGICAL WORKINGS

Red Powder: A Philter of Enlivening for Arcane Artifacts

This red powder has sanguine ingredients of a primal nature and is used for drawing life force into magical artifacts, tools, and relics of lore. Almost all of the plant ingredients are substitutes for or symbolic of blood. Sorcerers also add real blood to this powder, especially menstrual blood, which is known for its occult power. Through the generative forces of blood, we can create, enliven, and awaken magical objects, such as

*awakening the spirit within a poppet. Adding the sorcerer's own blood
can create a powerfully connected casting powder, which can be used to
activate the kamea.*

*This powder with its martial properties can also be used to lay the
boundaries of powerful protective barriers. It connects with the powerful
draconic currents of Earth, the serpent fire that provides light to the
underworld. It may be used to seal rites of oath making and for personal
protection when working curses and other aggressive or dark magic.*

- Bloodroot (*Sanguinaria canadensis*): The ground rootstock
  erects an intense protective barrier and is symbolic of blood.
- Dragon's blood resin: This deep red resin harvested from
  various plant species is a magical catalyst and potentiator of
  arcane formulas.
- Iron powder: As the blood of Earth, this powder imparts
  telluric currents into the formula and seals the other
  ingredients, along with the blood of the sorcerer.
- Red ocher: This clay earth pigment is a primal symbol of blood,
  used for reddening oracular skulls and bones and the casting
  of protective circles. Red ocher contains ferric oxide, which is
  basically rusted metal.
- Red sandalwood (*Pterocarpus santalinus*): The powdered
  heartwood of this tree conducts high spiritual vibrations and
  is used for the consecration and empowerment of magical
  objects.
- Yarrow (*Achillea millefolium*): Known as woundwort, this plant
  was used as a styptic on the battlefield, and thus it corresponds
  to blood and the energy of Mars. It acts as a container for
  energy, synergizing the other ingredients.

Combine all ingredients in equal parts, creating a fine powder.

Most people will not find these ingredients growing natively, except
for yarrow. Fortunately, they can all be acquired from your local herbalist, health food store, or metaphysical shop. Red ocher can also be found
online as it is sold as a pigment. Iron powder can be found anywhere

there is old rusty metal. The part you want can be carefully filed off and collected.

❦

Casting Powder for Circles, Sigils, and Dusting

This recipe creates a multipurpose powder for spell casting, drawing magical symbols, or sprinkling on enchanted objects. It can be used to create magical boundaries that can be used to keep forces within or alternatively to keep unwanted energies from entering. It contains ingredients to enhance power, manifest and draw forces, summon spirits, and empower symbols. It could be used for containment spells, unblocking, blessing, cleansing, and fortification of protection. Many of these herbs are magical catalysts used to empower any working.

- Belladonna (*Atropa belladonna*): *Atropa* brings Saturnian powers of crystallization and manifestation. It opens the gateways and the chakras, expanding awareness, and creates an aura of secrecy and shadow.
- Dragon's blood resin: This resin adds power and potency to any magical working, incorporating the fiery protection of Mars and the magical spirit of dragons.
- Master root (*Imperatoria ostruthium*) or High John the Conqueror root (*Ipomoea jalapa*): These roots, shaved to a fine powder, are used for their powers of commanding and mastery.
- Solomon's seal (*Polygonatum odoratum*): This plant is a magical catalyst for elemental energy and planetary powers and empowers sigils and seals. It is an herb of offering and manifestation, used to activate magical glyphs and sigils.
- Vervain (*Verbena officinalis*): A quintessential herb of enchantment, *Verbena* is used for its ability to empower magical objects and summon spirits. Vervain is a multipurpose magical catalyst.
- Yarrow (*Achillea millefolium*): *Achillea* creates a boundary and a vessel for the energy through its properties of sealing and

containment. It strengthens the perimeter of the aura and the magic circle, allowing it to constrict or expand as needed. Technically not psychoactive, yarrow is used by shamans to protect the body while journeying. Taken as an infusion, it cleanses the system, which is beneficial before fasting.

A binding agent—such as cornstarch, cascarilla (powdered eggshells), red brick dust, or red ocher—added to the powder mix confers its own protective, containing, and blessing properties. This sprinkling powder contains the energies within the symbol, circle, or object and can be dusted or blown over an altar prior to ritual. When placed in a cross formation, it acts as a portable crossroads and can be carried for magic while traveling. This is meant to be an all-purpose powder for feeding charms, activating talismans, and establishing one's power over an area. Its components make this a powerful offering or feeding powder for charm bags and magical objects. It can also be blown to the wind to carry a spell, requiring the ingredients to be ground as finely as possible. The action of pulverizing will further imbue this philter with one's focused power.

❧

Containment Mixture

This formula uses herbs of binding to stop a target from succeeding in their private pursuits of interfering in your own situation. It can be used in hexes of entropy, which weigh the target down, restricting their abilities and keeping them from making progress. For individuals working against you, it can be used to bind their actions. Alternatively, it can be used to seal dark energies within a cursed object that cannot be exorcised so that their influence is nullified, allowing the object to be safely removed. Harmful or haunted objects can be bound and taken away from those they are affecting for later removal and releasing.

- Agrimony (*Agrimonia eupatoria*): Provides precise protection within a designated area; seals energy within the target.
- Ashes: Holds energy within its boundary. Just as a circle of salt keeps thing out, ashes keep them in (used as a base for powder).

- Barberry (*Berberis vulgaris*): Blocks the way and closes the roads.
- Bindweed (*Convolvulus arvensis*), woody nightshade (*Solanum dulcamara*): Binds.
- Devil's shoestrings (*Nolina lindheimeriana*): Binds enemies by restricting their actions (used as a powder).
- Knotgrass (*Polygonum aviculare*): Restricts and binds, tying up a situation; used in entanglement charms.

Combine the ingredients in equal parts. It is important that all of the ingredients are ground as finely as possible to ensure an unbroken line when pouring the powder to draw boundaries and protective circles. Talc or cornstarch can also be used as a base for the mixture, to thicken it and make pouring easier.

❧

Ink of the Green Devil

The green devil is the adversarial side of nature, a Saturnian spirit representing what is wild and untamable. As green practitioners, we seek to connect with this power. The following recipe creates an ink or dye that can be used for imbuing objects with the verdant power of the Old One. The ink is created by making an alcohol extract or tincture of the desired plants. The resulting ink is dark green due to the chlorophyll. Chlorophyll is involved in photosynthesis and is synonymous with the blood of plants. It is particularly suited for the green witch.

- Fresh plant material
- 1 cup vodka
- 2–3 tsp. gum arabic

For this formula we are making a concentrated tincture, to extract the pigments from the plant material, and thickening it with gum arabic. The recipe makes one cup of ink, which is actually quite a bit. You can cut the recipe down if you like. The more plant material you add to the alcohol, and the more times you infuse it with fresh herbs, the darker it will be.

Put fresh plant material in a jar and cover with vodka; allow to macerate until a dark green color is achieved. Adding additional fresh plant material will create a darker color. Put the macerated plant material in a double boiler on low heat, add gum arabic, and stir thoroughly. Heating the mixture will dissolve the gum arabic, which improves the consistency of the ink.

The ink can be used for drawing plant spirit glyphs, sigils, and magical alphabets. It can also be employed for adding verdant hues to bones and skulls and for decorating and enlivening vessels for plant familiars and other nature spirits. In addition to writing, the tincture can be used as a wash for spell papers by applying a light coating and allowing it to dry before use. I typically use baneful herbs such as belladonna and datura in my magical inks, which are appropriate for the green devil. Other plants with an affinity to natural magic and the lord of the hunt could be incorporated, such as cinquefoil for success and mastery, centaury as a patron of herbalists, and master of the woods (*Asperula odorata*) for its commanding properties and connection to the lord of the wildwood.

Antidotes

- Activated charcoal is a safe and natural remedy taken for poisoning and overdose. Its porous surface area easily binds to toxins. It is typically taken as a drink mixed with water.
- Atropine is an antimuscarinic that reacts with the toxic muscarine found in trace amounts in *Amanita muscaria*. Atropine is also used as an antidote to foxglove poisoning.
- Belladonna (*Atropa belladonna*) has been used to treat opiate overdose and muscarinic mushroom poisoning (Voogelbreinder 2009, 97).
- Caffeine counteracts tropane alkaloid poisoning by reducing sedation and increasing acetylcholine activity. It is a central nervous system stimulant.

- Foxglove (*Digitalis* spp.) tincture was used as a traditional antidote for wolfsbane; there is no modern antidote for wolfsbane poisoning. Foxglove is a powerful emetic and stimulant.
- Lobelia (*Lobelia inflata*) was traditionally used for its purgative effects to treat poisoning. It can act as a stimulant or a depressant, easing nervous tension and panic.
- Mugwort (*Artemisia vulgaris*) is an antidote for opium poisoning (Voogelbreinder 2009, 92–93).
- Nicotine acts as an agonist, stimulating nicotinic acetylcholine receptors to produce a response countering the effects of the anticholinergic syndrome produced by tropane alkaloids.
- Physostigmine is a naturally occurring cholinergic found in the Calabar bean (*Physostigma venenosum*), a West African vine. It reverses the inhibition process of anticholinergics like the tropane alkaloids; however, its use is controversial due to its side effects, and it is reserved for the most serious cases of poisoning.

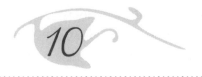

10

The Other Garden
Cultivation and Harvesting

*B*aneful herbs are wild and uncultivated. They have remained alongside humanity this entire time without being "domesticated" like common garden plants. Although some of them show up in ornamental gardens and churchyards, they maintain their untamable spirit. This is great for magic, but not so much for cultivation. Baneful herbs are used to proliferating on their own in the wild and grow willingly for humans with a little coaxing. Some baneful herbs require long periods of cold before they germinate. Others do better with growth hormones to kick-start the germination process. Often growing in waste areas, hedgerows, and other in-between places, baneful herbs thrive without human intervention. This chapter includes tips on starting seeds and caring for plants once they are mature. There is information covering all parts of each plant's life cycle, from germination and growth to harvesting.

✸

Belladonna (*Atropa belladonna*)

Certain seeds require cold soaking to successfully germinate. Cold stratification removes the layer of chemicals present around some seeds that prevent germination. This is achieved by putting the seeds through a period of cold soaking to gradually remove these chemicals by mimicking the melting of snow.

The seeds are placed in a container with water and refrigerated for a period of two to four weeks, during which the water is changed daily. I use distilled water and make a little pouch using a coffee filter so the seeds don't run out when you change the water. The bottom or back of the refrigerator is the coldest and has worked for me.

It is said that belladonna has a germination rate of 60 to 70 percent. Seeds over a year old have a better germination rate than brand-new seeds. I have had a germination rate of 90 percent with older seeds in two to three weeks using this method. The berries contain seeds and can be planted directly, or the seeds sown on the winter solstice, providing them with the necessary periods of cold and warm.

Belladonna prefers full or partial shade. Direct hot sunlight puts stress on the plant, causing it to produce higher amounts of alkaloids. It grows best in soil that is calcareous, meaning it contains lime. It is slightly alkaline, chalky, or containing limestone. This can be achieved if soil is too acidic by purchasing lime or powdered limestone from your local garden center. If you are growing in pots, pieces of chalk or lime can be placed over drainage holes in the bottom of the container.

The alkaloid content is the highest when the berries are forming and the lowest when the plant is in flower, although this is often happening simultaneously. The plant blooms from late spring (end of June) until the early fall (September–October). Seasons that are exceptionally hot and dry produce a higher alkaloid content than seasons that are mild.

Experiments on water stress and nitrogen fertilization have also yielded higher alkaloid contents for pharmaceutical production (Baricevic et al.).

The leaves can be harvested earlier in mature plants, usually starting in May or June; however, first-year harvesting should be postponed until July or August. This should be done sustainably in the first year so that the plant is not unnecessarily stressed. Second-year plants can be harvested in their entirety in May and June, being cut down to one inch above the ground, and will then yield a second harvest in the fall.

In the first year, the plant grows to 1.5 to 3 feet and in subsequent years reaches 4 to 6 feet.

Harvesting Belladonna

While I personally harvest leaves, flowers, and berries throughout the season for their many different uses, the entire plant can be harvested in the fall. This includes the roots, which are then dried or preserved in alcohol to create powerful plant spirit fetishes. Belladonna is a perennial and can be cut down, leaving the roots to come back for many years to come.

If using the plant for medicinal purposes or when the alkaloid content is of concern, it is important to dry the leaves quickly in direct sunlight in a well-ventilated area or in a dehydrator. The more faded the plant material, the lower the alkaloid content.

Black Mandrake (*Mandragora autumnalis*)

Black or autumn mandrake is native to southern Europe, the Mediterranean, and parts of the Middle East. It blooms in the fall, instead of in spring like its cousin *Mandragora officinarum,* and its flowers are a soft violet color.

Mandrake is characteristically difficult to germinate, which is no surprise for such an elusive and mysterious plant. Germination is irregular, but for some lucky people, it seems to sprout with no hesitation. The cold soaking method can also be used to help germination. Alternatively, the seeds can be planted in peat pellets, which are sold at your local garden center. The pellets come in trays, and when water is added, the little disks expand, creating a convenient little greenhouse in which to start your seeds. Once planted, the entire tray can be placed in the refrigerator, covered, for four to six weeks. The soil should be kept moist, but not wet, and out of direct sunlight. Patience is needed with this plant as it is slow to come up.

The plant can be potted so that it can be overwintered indoors. The pot should be deeper than it is wide; three to four feet deep is ideal to provide space for the root. For black mandrake, peat can be added to the soil to increase acidity. A mixture of peat, sand, and loam can be used in a ratio of 2:2:1 to provide proper drainage. The soil should be kept moist, as the plant will go dormant if dry, but not overly wet. It should only be watered when the soil is dry to the touch.

It should be fertilized regularly using an organic fertilizer such as kelp solution. When watering, avoid watering the leaves so that they do not succumb to mold. The plant prefers partial sun to shade. When potted, the plant may be overwintered indoors; however, it should not be watered while the plant is in its dormant stage. If transplanting outdoors, be careful with the roots, as they become brittle to promote propagation.

Root cuttings may be taken after the first season of growth. The root is divided into one- to two-inch pieces. The root pieces are then cut horizontally across the top and at an angle on the bottom. The root cuttings are dipped in rooting hormone, such as an infusion of willow bark. They are then planted in a soil and sand mixture. The root tubers can be divided in late autumn and planted for the following spring.

🌿

White Mandrake
(Mandragora officinarum)

The white or spring mandrake has greenish-white to soft violet-blue flowers. It has a shorter stalk with a taproot that grows quickly. The plant is usually less than a foot tall, but the root can grow up to four feet long over consecutive seasons. The same seed-starting techniques can be used for both black and white mandrake.

Remember, the seeds can be slow to germinate, sometimes sprouting after six months to a year, so long as they are kept moist and out of the sun. Fresh seeds may be planted in cactus mix and placed in a warm but shaded area. Fresh seeds will sprout after eight months. Cold soaking reduces the germination time for dry seeds. They can be planted in sandy soil and watered daily. They should be kept warm but out of direct sunlight.

White mandrake prefers rocky, alkaline soil. Limestone or ground oyster shells may be mixed into the soil, while coarse sand or pumice can be used to increase drainage by building up around the crown of the plant. This plant grows best when roots have room to grow, so if planting in a pot for easy harvest, make sure it has enough depth. The roots become brittle, so take care when transplanting or propagating. Watering the plants beforehand helps soften and release the soil around the root. It is very easy to break the root when digging it out of the ground, so many people choose to pot their mandrakes.

It is best to transplant the plant outdoors when it is in its vegetative phase, not in dormancy. This can be done in early spring when the plant will keep its leaves for a couple more months before summer dormancy. To help the plant acclimate to the outdoors, a hole can be dug and the entire pot placed in the ground in the desired area until the plant is ready. I would give it a week to become acclimated.

Dormancy and Propagation

Mandrakes typically go dormant throughout the season. They often do so at inconvenient times, seemingly following their own schedule. Oftentimes, they will go dormant during the peak of the summer heat, often corresponding to the dog days. They also go dormant in the winter, even when kept in a greenhouse. When the plant goes dormant, its leaves begin to yellow and brown before falling off. The root continues to thrive beneath the soil, where the majority of the plant's mass lives. It is important to avoid dormancy from occurring for an entire season to get the mandrake to fruit.

In an attempt to avoid dormancy from occurring, make sure the plant does not receive too much or too little water, watering only when the soil is dry. Fertilize regularly using a liquid kelp fertilizer. Also avoid extreme temperatures of hot or cold. Dormancy is a natural part of plants' life cycle. If dormancy happens, don't worry and be patient: the plant will come back. The most important thing to remember when the plant is in dormancy is not to overwater it! Too much water will cause the root to rot. Water less during the winter when the plant is dormant and only when soil is dry; water less than you normally would when the plant is producing leaves. Drainage is also very important during this time.

Mandrakes are self-propagating, growing small extensions off the main root that eventually break off and start a new plant. The roots are brittle so that they can easily detach. After the first season of growth, the plant can be propagated by root cuttings. Cuttings are taken from smaller parts off the main root. Take a cutting that is two inches long by slicing the upper part of the cutting horizontally and the lower part at an angle. Dip the cutting in a rooting hormone or willow bark infusion. Plant in a covered location in sandy soil. Divide the tubers in the autumn and plant for the following spring.

Harvesting the Mandrake

There is a large body of tradition and folklore surrounding the harvesting of the mandrake.

1. Traditionally, a plant is selected between the winter solstice and vernal equinox, when the roots are hibernating and contain the plant's vital energy. A clockwise circle is traced around the plant, and the intention is stated, while offerings are made.
2. Right after the new moon, before it begins waxing, the root is carefully exhumed, lower leaves are removed, and a ritual blade is used to carve the root into a more humanoid shape. Traditionally, the root would represent the opposite sex of the practitioner; however, it is often androgynous. Care is taken during the carving process, and only mature roots (three to four years old) are carved.
3. The root is reinterred and left in the soil for an entire moon cycle. The practitioner regularly visits the plant for watering and libations containing small amounts of milk or blood. During this time, the carved parts of the root heal. With regular offerings and invocations, the plant spirit is empowered and called into the root.
4. At the end of the lunar cycle, the root is dug up and allowed to dry,

which is a slow process that can take a couple of months. It is traditionally appropriate to fumigate the drying root with the smoke of vervain.

❀

Black Henbane (*Hyoscyamus niger*), White Henbane (*Hyoscyamus albus*)

Henbane produces numerous seeds, which can be surface-sown in late spring or early summer. They are often quick to germinate, depending on the species and their origin. Seeds may be cold-soaked for two weeks, after which they will germinate within ten days. If germination does not occur within three to four weeks, a cooling period of two to four weeks may be needed. GA3 hormone or gibberellic acid can also help with germination.

Henbane grown in pots is often stunted unless a large pot is used. It should be transplanted to its final location outside when the seedlings reach two inches tall. It is important to transplant before the plants begin to flower; this avoids stunting their growth. The plants can be planted in clusters because they form taproots, which do not spread out. Henbane can be planted in sunny areas in well-drained soil that is sandy and alkaline, but like other nightshades, it will temporarily wilt in the heat. Henbane is used to growing in warm climates and likes growing in poor soil and in cracks and crevices, preferring this to overly moist fertile soil.

Be careful not to overwater henbane because it is prone to damping off. The leaves will mold if you get them wet when watering, so water the soil beneath the plant only. Water only when the soil is dry. It can be watered more when flowering. Fertilize it by placing compost in a ring around the plant extending outside its drip line. An organic foliage fertilizer, such as fish emulsion, may be used and is sprayed under the leaves in the early part of the day. Henbane is a hardy perennial and does not require extra care. One of the easiest ways to kill henbane is to overnurture it. Overwatering is common.

※

Egyptian Henbane (*Hyoscyamus muticus*)

This variety of henbane has fleshy succulent leaves, and the flowers range from a pinkish white to darker violet with veins. Valued as a pharmaceutical crop and in medicinal herbalism for its higher alkaloid content, *Hyoscyamus muticus* contains an alkaloid content of 5 percent in dry plant matter with smaller concentrations in the roots and stems.

Egyptian henbane thrives in a hot, sunny environment with low humidity. Surface-sow seeds and keep in a sunny, warm place, above 50 degrees. Viable Egyptian henbane seeds germinate readily, especially when soaked in a germination formula. It is important to keep humidity to a minimum, growing in full sun in well-draining soil. Like other varieties of henbane, it likes to grow on the wayside in poor soil, along roadsides and in old buildings. Sandy soil or chalky loam is also preferable to extremely rich soils. The plants do respond well to regular watering.

Harvesting Henbane

Henbane leaves can be collected when the plant is in full flower, starting at the beginning of summer. The seeds should be gathered in their capsules at the end of summer before their capsules split, spilling hundreds of seeds around the plant. For replanting, the seeds should be dried in the sun; for medicinal purposes, they can be dried in an oven or dehydrator. Henbane seeds are said to remain viable for hundreds of years. The capsules, which are striking in appearance, can be collected and saved and used on altars, in wreaths, and for spell work.

※

Opium Poppy (*Papaver somniferum*)

This annual plant can be fragile and demanding; however, sowing in the fall will provide needed resistance, giving the hardiest results. They can be planted in late winter to early spring. I live in a cooler spring climate (zone 5b–6a) and have planted my poppies in late April with good results. Poppies are best grown outdoors, left undisturbed. Starting them indoors and transplanting them often is too traumatic for these sensitive plants. They are averse to any kind of root distur- bance and prefer a neutral to slightly alkaline soil, rich in nutrients, humus, and lime.

The seeds are surface-sown: work the soil slightly, sprinkle the seeds on the surface, and tamp them down. They will germinate when the weather becomes temperate, consistently reaching 55 to 60 degrees. The leaves become serrated and are thicker and not as delicate as those of the California poppy. Once the seedlings are one to two inches tall, they can be thinned. Keeping them in close proximity will result in the plants growing taller and weedier.

Continue to weed them to avoid competition and water regularly. As they mature, they become top-heavy and should be protected from strong wind. I have planted mine along a small garden fence to provide a wind shield. They prefer full sun to partial shade.

Harvesting Poppy

The leaves may be collected in the summer, when the fruit capsules are maturing. The capsules can be collected for seeds and dried for use in ritual. Cut the stem a few inches down from the pod and allow the pod to dry fully intact, sealing the seeds within. The crown of the pod will open and spill seeds when the mature pod begins to brown. Collect the seeds just before this stage and save them, or let the plant reseed itself. The collection of opium latex from the poppy, which has been used in medicine for centuries, is illegal in the United States and other coun- tries. Tinctures and other analgesic medicines can be made using the seedpods. The leaves can be removed from the stems and dried to add to incense and smoking blends.

THE SACRED DATURAS

Moonflower (*Datura inoxia*)

Also called toloache, angel's trumpet, and prickly burr, this variety of *Datura* is native to the United States, Mexico, and Central and South America and is an annual or short-lived perennial shrub. It branches off into many divisions, and at each branching, a white, trumpet-shaped flower opens. The flower then turns into a low-hanging globular seed-pod covered in short spines. The flowers usually open in the evening and fade within a day. The leaves have a soft green color and are more oval shaped. They are not serrated like those of other varieties. The seeds are a medium brown color and contain higher amounts of alkaloids than those of some of the other varieties.

Jimson Weed (*Datura stramonium*)

Also called devil's apple, this variety grows across Europe and North America and is responsible for the Jamestown poisoning. *D. stramonium* was an ingredient in witches' flying ointments and is known for its distinct, intoxicating smell, which it releases at night to attract pollinating moths. Its white flowers are more lobed and pointed, blooming from early summer into midautumn. The stems are green compared to the purple stems of *D. stramonium* var. *tatula*. The fruits form more upright and have longer and sharper spines, containing dark brown-black seeds.

Desert Thorn Apple (*Datura discolor*)

A relatively rare native plant of the American Southwest and Mexico, *D. discolor* has similar ritual uses to toloache, as they both grow in the same area. The flowers are white with purple, blooming at night, releasing their sweet scent. The seedpods are thorny and pendulous and contain black seeds.

⚛

Indian Thorn Apple (*Datura metel*)

In ancient Sanskrit, this plant was called *unmata,* meaning "divine inebriation." It's an annual herbaceous plant, with slightly serrated, soft, light-green leaves, and is thought to have originated in northern India. The flowers range from violet to yellow and white, often growing double or triple within the same bloom (Rätsch 2005, 203). It now grows throughout Central and South America and the Caribbean. *Datura metel* contains the highest concentration of scopolamine out of the genus.

⚛

Sacred Datura (*Datura wrightii*)

Native to the American Southwest, sacred datura has been used traditionally by indigenous people as a healing plant and for its visionary effects. It has large white trumpet-shaped flowers with widely spaced lobes. The leaves are soft green, ovate, and deeply veined. Unlike other daturas, *D. wrightii* grows close to the ground, spreading out like a vine.

Growing and Harvesting Datura

All varieties of *Datura* that I have had experience planting seem to germinate within two to eight weeks. Some varieties are more irregular than others, such as *D. stramonium,* with some seeds sprouting within one to two weeks and others sprouting subsequently. Germination occurs at warmer temperatures, and greenhouse germination is very successful. As an annual, it seems to do well when planted in a large pot, although it will often wilt on hot days. They prefer warm sunny locations in rich soil that is kept warm and moist. They take well to compost fertilizer as well as manure. Plant out when seedlings reach two to three inches.

The leaves can be gathered when the plant is in full bloom and used in preparations for both medicine and magic. Harvesting too young of a plant may result in too much hyoscyamine or atropine and not enough scopolamine. The leaves and seeds lend themselves well to oils and ointments for their pain-relieving properties. The leaves are traditionally dried and smoked with tobacco for their intoxicating effects. The flowers can also be collected. The leaves, flowers, and seeds all contain the medicinal properties of the plant. Once they begin to close, the flowers can be carefully slid off the plant without interfering with the production of seedpods. The flowers can be pressed for drying and used in spell work to incorporate the magical properties of this plant.

The seedpods should not be harvested until mature. Some people will wait until they just begin to split or turn brown. I take them when they are still green and about the size of a golf ball. After this point, the seeds are mature, and they will continue to ripen and often split on their own off the plant. It is important that the seedpods be dried completely in a place with low moisture. The seedpods should be split open to dry; if there is too much moisture, the seeds will mold and will be rendered unviable. The pods may also be used for their alkaloid content and can be stored separately from the seeds and reserved for ritual uses. Their thorns provide a powerful sympathetic magic. Once the seeds are properly dried, they can be kept for many years and remain viable. Test results after thirty-nine years have shown seeds that were still 90 percent viable (Heiser 1969).

MONKSHOOD AND WOLFSBANE

Monkshood and wolfsbane are both members of the Ranunculaceae or buttercup family. Their names are often used interchangeably, and in medieval references, both plants are considered essentially the same, magically and chemically. But though they both belong to the genus *Aconitum,* they are distinct species with characteristic differences. For one, monkshood is distinguished from wolfsbane by it blue-purple flowers.

❦

Monkshood (*Aconitum napellus*)

Monkshood is a perennial that can live for many years. It generally does not flower in its first year. The leaves may be harvested in late summer by cutting down the stem before the plant dies back in the fall. It has dark-green, intricately lobed leaves. It is a woodland plant, growing in damp undergrowth and often found near streams. It is native to western and central Europe and can be found growing in mountainous areas at high elevations.

Monkshood seeds can be slow to germinate and often require a period of cold. They are best sown in the fall; however, they can be cold stratified. To do so, wrap them in a damp paper towel, seal the towel in a ziplock plastic bag, and place the bag in the freezer. Doing this will mimic the cold winter temperature necessary to awaken the seeds. Monkshood requires two to three weeks of warm moisture followed by three to five months of cold. An easy way to achieve this is to plant the seeds in a seed tray, leave the tray at room temperature for two to three weeks, then place the tray in the refrigerator with its cover on for three to five months. After this period the seeds will begin to germinate. Once the seeds sprout, they can be planted in a pot; when the seedlings are large enough, they can be transplanted to individual pots and kept in a cold frame over the winter. Monkshood thrives in moist calcareous soil containing chalk or limestone. Compost made from fallen leaves or manure can be used. These plants prefer semishade and will thrive in sunny spots only if the soil is kept moist.

⚘

Wolfsbane (*Aconitum lycoctonum*)

A close relative of monkshood, wolfsbane can be distinguished by its greenish-yellow to off-white flowers. The "hood" on this flower is more elongated than that of monkshood. It also grows in damp, shady, wooded areas and in open fields. It blooms from June to August and is a perennial. The plant can be grown in partial sun to partial shade.

Its seeds, like those of other aconites, are sometimes difficult to germinate and can be coaxed similarly to monkshood seeds. Wrap the seeds in a damp paper towel and keep in an open ziplock plastic bag for four weeks out of direct sunlight. The bag can then be sealed and placed in the freezer for six weeks. Or just plant the seeds in a pot in the fall and keep the pot outdoors over the winter. If you live in an area that gets a lot of snow, the seeds can be potted and kept in a covered area or direct-sown and covered with mulch.

Harvesting Monkshood and Wolfsbane

These plants are often stored according to their growth cycles. Their active constituents remain viable for up to one year. The flowers can be collected and dried for use in spells and ritual or used fresh to create flower essences for safely working with these toxic plants. It is important to wear gloves when working with the fresh plant material, as it remains extremely toxic until dried; the roots are especially poisonous. The old root—the previous year's portion—may be harvested when the plant dies down in the fall. The leaves and flowers can be harvested when the plant is in flower and dried before use. Although aconite is used in traditional Chinese medicine (TCM), it is not recommended that this plant be ingested or used topically. Aconitine poisoning is one of the most common causes of poisoning in TCM.

※

Poison Hemlock
(Conium maculatum)

Poison hemlock is a biennial that grows in moist areas, often along streams and rivers. It is easily confused with water hemlock, which is just as poisonous if not more so. Hemlock has also been confused with several other plants, such as wild carrot and parsley, which has resulted in accidental poisoning. It resembles Queen Anne's lace, which grows abundantly in my area. Hemlock often grows taller than Queen Anne's lace, and its flowers are all white, while Queen Anne's lace has the characteristic dark flower in the center, representing a drop of blood. Hemlock stems are smooth and bear the "mark of Cain," dark-purple spots along the stem. The stems of Queen Anne's lace are green and hairy.

Poison hemlock grows in a rosette during its first year and sends up a stalk in the second year. The seeds germinate from early spring to late summer, preferring cooler temperatures. They can be surface-sown at room temperature, barely covered with soil, and will germinate in two weeks.

Hemlock is an extremely poisonous plant, and care should be taken when handling the fresh plant material. Like many alkaloid-containing plants, the warmer the weather, the higher the alkaloid content. The alkaloids travel an upward path throughout the season and are initially more concentrated in the roots. They move subsequently throughout the plant over its growth cycle, and by the end of the season, the seeds have a higher alkaloid content. Coniine is the primary alkaloid in poison hemlock and is present at 0.5 percent by weight. Just a few leaves are enough to kill a person. Much of the alkaloids are destroyed when heating or boiling the plant and do not remain in the dried plant material.

Black Hellebore (*Helleborus niger*)

This cold-hardy plant is one of the first to bloom in late winter to early spring, which is where it gets the name Lenten rose. There are many varieties of hellebore, including many hybrid varieties that have been cultivated for their unique beauty. They are an evergreen perennial plant in the Ranunculaceae family. While some varieties have flowers that look black, this variety has flowers that are whitish green. The flowers are thick and leathery, almost leaflike.

For the seeds to germinate, they must go through a period of warm and then cold treatment. The seeds should be planted and kept at room temperature with constant humidity for four to six weeks. They do well in small indoor greenhouses and seed-starting containers with a plastic cover, which retain warmth and moisture. A waterproof heating pad for plants can also be used to provide heat from the bottom. After this period, the temperature is lowered gradually: the seeds are first placed in the refrigerator for one to two weeks and can then be transferred to the freezer for six weeks. If the cooling period was long enough, the seeds should germinate once taken out of the freezer. Sometimes the seeds will not germinate until the following spring.

Once the seedlings are about two inches tall, they can be transplanted. These are woodland plants and prefer dappled shade; they will wilt in direct sunlight. They prefer deep, well-drained, fertile soil, with no competition from nearby trees. Sometimes they can take up to two years before they bloom, but they keep their green leaves throughout most of the year. Mulch can be built up around the plants to protect them from harsh winters. Although the plants self-sow, they can be propagated by root division in late summer.

The dead leaves should be picked off regularly to prevent disease. Both the leaves and flowers can be collected when the plant is in flower and dried for later use. The leaves and flowers are thick and succulent, taking time to dry, but once dry, they can be kept for long periods.

❦

Foxglove (*Digitalis purpurea*)

Foxglove is a biennial plant in the Plantaginaceae family and once belonged to the figwort family (Scrophulariaceae). This woodland plant is native to western Europe, western and central Asia, and northwest Africa. It is a traditional cottage garden plant and is still commonly grown as an ornamental. It prefers a silica-rich, acidic, loamy soil (fertile soil containing clay, sand, and composted leaves). Foxglove tolerates shade and will also grow in full sun; however, it does not like extreme heat. When planting it in a sunny spot, keep it on the north side. Alternatively, when planting it in a southern exposure, keep it in the shade to avoid extreme heat.

The seeds germinate readily and can be sown at room temperature. The seeds are tiny and numerous. They can be surface-sown and should be kept moist. If the seeds are started early enough, the plant will reseed itself during the same season. It typically grows a rosette of leaves the first season and sends up its stalks the second. If you have purchased a plant from a garden center, it should flower the same year. The entire stalk can be cut down in the summer and dried to save the flowers. This also helps send energy back to the root system so that it can protect itself from harsh winter. In previous years I have cut down one stalk, and several smaller ones have returned in its place before the end of the season.

❦

Mugwort (*Artemisia vulgaris*), Wormwood (*Artemisia absinthium*)

Mugwort belongs to the *Artemisia* genus and is native to North America, Europe, and Asia. It is a hardy perennial that is cold tolerate and propagates itself by sending out creeping rhizomes. This bushy perennial can reach five to seven feet in height and will spread out wherever it has room. Once established, it can be propagated by dividing the rhizomes in early spring.

The seeds need light to germinate and should be sprinkled and patted into moist soil. Mugwort prefers rich, moist soil and full sun. The seeds can be planted at the winter solstice or in early spring. If planted indoors, they should be kept at cold temperatures for a couple of weeks. The leaves can be collected throughout the season once the plant is established. They are soft and fuzzy and have a wide spectrum of ritual and medicinal uses. Collecting the leaves before the plant begins to flower will ensure the highest oil content. The root can be harvested in the fall.

Wormwood is also a member of the *Artemisia* genus and works synergistically with mugwort. It is also a hardy perennial and grows abundantly across Europe and North America. Wormood has tiny seeds, which can be surface-sown because they need light to germinate. The seeds can be sprinkled and patted into moist soil that is kept hydrated by misting. Keep out of full sun and keep at room temperature until germination occurs.

Wormwood is an allelopathic plant, meaning it releases chemical compounds from its roots into the soil that suppress the growth of or even kill nearby plants. It can be grown in containers or kept separately from other plants. This abundant plant produces indefinitely and can be harvested continually once established. Often reaching a height of four to five feet when planted in the ground, it can be cut back during its second year and will replenish itself that season.

Aztec Tobacco (*Nicotiana rustica*)

The tobacco plant is a member of the Solanaceae family and, like tomatoes, can be easy to grow. It can be grown in large amounts as a natural alternative to commercially grown tobacco, having less chemicals than manufactured cigarettes. *Nicotiana rustica* has, however, a higher nicotine content than other varieties, such as *N. tabacum* or *N. virginiana*.

Tobacco seeds are very tiny, even smaller than poppy seeds, and should be planted by surface sowing. They can be sown outside after the danger of frost is passed. The seeds can be started in seed boxes or trofts and kept in a partially shaded area that is shielded from rain.

The soil should be kept moist, and keeping seed boxes in partial shade will prevent the sun from drying out the soil and ensure that the seeds do not blow away. The seedlings can be transplanted when they have reached two inches. When ready for transplant, the seedlings can be moved to an area that receives full sunlight.

Tobacco prefers nutrient-rich soils; using compost to fertilize the soil or as the sole planting medium is beneficial. The plants will reach 2 feet in diameter and 1.5 feet high. *N. rustica* can be spaced closer together than other varieties. While tobacco is sensitive to cold, it can be grown in a wide range of areas, including the United Kingdom and United States.

Harvesting and Preparation

The oldest method of harvesting tobacco is to cut the entire plant at its base before flowering, which typically happens in July and August, and hang it to dry. The plant is ready to harvest when the tips of the leaves begin to turn yellow.

Individual leaves can also be harvested and tied into bundles, which are then hung to dry in the sun or in a dark and well-ventilated area, such as a barn, shed, or garage. Leaves can be harvested throughout the season, and the flower tops cut off to increase leaf production. Tobacco leaves are typically cured for four to eight weeks before use. Aging tobacco reduces the sugar content, giving it a light and smooth flavor.

HOMEMADE PESTICIDES

Soap and Oil Sprays

These sprays work against insects as well as molds and fungi. Many of the plants listed in this book are prone to predation by a variety of insects. The leaves of the nightshades are also susceptible to different molds and mildews. These blends will help prevent and treat these conditions. They are effective against their targets but are safe for the environment, pets, and wildlife. As insecticides, they work by disrupting an insect's hormones, preventing an insect from feeding, or coating the pores in an insect's exoskeleton, which essentially asphyxiates it. These recipes are all similar, consisting of a vegetable oil and mild liquid soap. A wide range of essential oils may also be incorporated for their anti-fungal and insecticidal properties. Use these sprays in the morning or evening before the heat of the day.

❧

Insect Repellent and Fungicide for Blight and Mildew

- 1 Tbsp. baking soda
- ½ tsp. mild detergent
- 2½ Tbsp. olive or other vegetable oil
- 1 gallon water

Mix and spray on foliage, shaking the mixture before use.

❧

Oil and Soap Spray

- 1 cup vegetable oil
- 1 Tbsp. liquid soap

Add two tablespoons of this mixture to one quart of water and spray on foliage. There are containers used to spray plant food or fertilizer that are hooked up to a garden hose and can be used to spray this repellent.

❧

Soap Spray

- 1½ tsp. mild liquid soap
- 1 qt. water

Mix and spray on foliage.

◥◣◥

Neem Oil Spray

- ❧ 2 tsp. neem oil
- ❧ 1 tsp. liquid soap
- ❧ 1 qt. water

Neem oil is found in seeds from the neem tree and is biodegradable and nontoxic to pets and wildlife. You can purchase a premixed spray at any garden center, or you can make your own from pure neem oil. The oil is a hormone disruptor as well as an antifeedant and effectively kills insects at all stages of life: adults, larvae, and eggs. It is also effective against mildew and fungal infections.

Insecticidal Nightshades

The alkaloids in the relatives of some of the very plants we are trying to protect are effective insecticides and vermicides. These nightshades have been used traditionally as pest control and are known for their effectiveness.

- **Tobacco leaf:** Some varieties of tobacco have been grown for their use as an insecticide. The nicotine alkaloids are effective against insects and other small pests. An infusion of the leaves is made by chopping the leaves and steeping them overnight in water and then straining and spraying on the foliage.
- **Tomato leaf:** The tomatine alkaloids are effective against aphids and other plant-feeding insects that can decimate a plant in a short amount of time. Steep two cups of chopped tomato leaves in one quart of water overnight. Strain and spray the mixture on the foliage.

Conclusion

$\mathcal{W}$e have explored these magical plants from a mythological, historical, and scientific perspective. We have heard their stories and traced their fantastic journeys to get a better understanding of the plant spirits themselves. To know their stories is to know the story of witchcraft, and how through an understanding of the natural world certain individuals have tapped into this ancient power. By exploring all of these different facets of each plant, we begin to get a sense for the personality of each particular spirit. This knowledge can aid us in our workings and bring deeper understanding to our interactions with the natural world.

By now there are probably a few plants that have called out to you. You may resonate with their mythos, their magical correspondences, or something more personal. It is this attraction that is your first sign that these spirits are trying to reach out to you. Tap into that connection and make it stronger. Learn everything you can about that specific plant spirit and see what insights arise with this new understanding.

Plant spirits are colorful, vibrant, and unique individuals. They interact with us all on a very individual basis. There are many ways to connect with a plant spirit, and once a rapport is established, you will come to understand the reason that you are drawn to this spirit.

The plants are really calling out to us during this tumultuous time, when social paradigms are shifting and the world as we know it is transforming before our eyes. There is a reason that these plants have returned to our conscious attention, and it is to help facilitate all of the change and growth that is happening.

The greatest lesson these plants teach us is that poison is not always what it seems. Sometimes the very thing that is the bane of our existence becomes the driving force that pushes us to the next level in our development. We need to remember the ancient concept of the *pharmaka,* a plant that is magic, medicine, and poison all in one. Poison is just another way of describing potency, and it is important to remember that what makes a plant poisonous is also what makes it medicinal. I'll leave you with the Paracelsian adage "the dose makes the poison," which challenged the belief that poisons were inherently toxic. It is this knowledge that will light the way as we walk the Poison Path.

Works Cited

Adams, James David Jr., and Cecilia Garcia. 2005. "The Advantages of Traditional Chumash Healing." *Evidence Based Complementary Alternative Medicine* 2, no. 1: 19–23.

Adams, James David Jr., and Xiaogang Wang. 2015. "Control of Pain with Topical Plant Medicines." *Asian Pacific Journal of Tropical Biomedicine* 5, no. 4: 268–73.

Agrippa, Heinrich Cornelius. 1533. *Three Books of Occult Philosophy.*

Ahrens, F. B. 1889. "Die alkaloide der Mandragora." *Justus Liebigs Annalen der Chemie* 25: 312–16.

Alizadeh, Anahita, Mohammad Moshiri, Javad Alizadeh, and Mahdi Balali-Mood. 2014. "Black Henbane and Its Toxicity: A Descriptive Review." *Avicenna Journal of Phytomedicine* 4, no. 5: 297–311.

Arena, J. M. 1974. *Poisoning: Toxicology-Symptoms-Treatments.* 3rd ed. Springfield, Ill.: Charles C. Thomas.

Arnett, Amy M. 1995. "Jimson Weed (*Datura stramonium*) Poisoning." *Clinical Toxicology Review.* Massachusetts Poison Control System 18, no. 3.

Baricevic, Dea, Andrej Umek, Samo Kreft, Branivoj Maticic, and Alenka Zupancic. 1999. "Effect of Water Stress and Nitrogen Fertilization on the Content of Hyoscyamine and Scopolamine in the Roots of Deadly Nightshade (*Atropa belladonna*)." *Environmental and Experimental Botany* 42:17–24.

Black Koltuv, Barbara. 1986. *The Book of Lilith.* York Beach, Maine: Nicholas-Hays.

Börsch-Haubold, Angelika. 2007. "Plant Hallucinogens as Magical Medicines." *Science in School: The European Journal for Science Teachers,* no. 4.

Borgia, Valentina, Michelle Carlin, and Jacopo Crezzini. 2016. "Poison, Plants and Paleolithic Hunters." *Quarternary International* 427:94–103.

Boyer, Corinne. 2017. *Plants of the Devil.* Rancho Boca de la Cañada del Pinole, Calif.: Three Hands Press.

Caton, Gary P. 2017. *Hermetica Tryptycha: The Mercury Elemental Year.* Auckland, New Zealand: Rubedo Press.

Church, Stephen, and Carol Church. 2009. "Harvesting & Making Specific Tinctures." The Herbarium (website).

Cordano, Hieronymous. 1551. *De subtilitate.* Venice: Gulielmum Rouillium.

Cox, P. A. 2010. "Nervous System and Behavioral Toxicology." In *Comprehensive Toxicology,* edited by Charlene A. McQueen. 2nd ed. Amsterdam, Netherlands: Elsevier.

Crystalinks. 2009. "Ancient Egyptian Medicine." Crystalinks website.

Datta, Animesh K., and Paul Rita. 2011. "An Updated Overview on Atropa belladonna." *International Research Journal of Pharmacy* 2, no. 11: 11–17.

DeKorne, Jim. 1994. *Psychedelic Shamanism: The Cultivation, Preparation and Use of Psychotropic Plants.* Yakima, Wash.: Breakout Productions.

Dominguez, Ivo Jr. 2016. *Practical Astrology for Witches and Pagans: Using the Planets and the Stars for Effective Spellwork, Rituals, and Magickal Work.* San Francisco: Weiser Books.

Draco, Melusine. 2017. *By Wolfsbane and Mandrake Root.* Hampshire, UK: Moon Books.

Elworthy, Fredrick Thomas. 1895. *The Evil Eye.* London: J. Murray.

EMA. 1998. "Atropa Belladonna: Summary Report." Committee for Veterinary Medicinal Products. European Agency for the Evaluation of Medicinal Products (EMA), Veterinary Medicine Evaluation Unit.

Faivre, Antoine. 2003. *The Eternal Hermes: From Greek God to Alchemical Magus.* Grand Rapids, Mich.: Phanes Press.

Farrer-Halls, Gill. 2005. *The Aromatherapy Bible.* New York: Sterling.

Folkard, Richard. 1884. *Plant Lore, Legends and Lyrics.* London: S. Low, Marston, Searle, and Rivington.

Frisvold, Nikolaj de Mattos. 2014. *Craft of the Untamed.* Oxford, UK: Mandrake.

Funayama, Shinji, and Geoffrey Cordell. 2015. *Alkaloids: A Treasury of Poisons and Medicines.* Cambridge, Mass.: Academic Press.

Furbee, Brent. 2009. "Neurotoxic Plants." Chap. 47 in *Clinical Neurotoxicology: Syndromes, Substances, Environments,* edited by Michael R. Dobbs. Amsterdam, Netherlands: Elsevier.

Green, Monica H. 2010. *The Trotula: An English Translation of the Medieval Compendium of Women's Medicine.* Philadelphia: University of Pennsylvania Press.

Grieve, M. 1971. *A Modern Herbal: The Medicinal, Culinary, Cosmetic and Folk-Lore of Herbs, Grasses, Fungi, Shrubs & Trees with All Their Modern Scientific Uses.* Vol. 1 (A–H). New York: Dover.

Harner, Michael J., ed. 1973. *Hallucinogens and Shamanism.* New York: Oxford University Press.

Hartlieb, Johannes. 2016. *Das Puch Aller Verpoten Kunst, Ungelaubens und der Zaubrey* (The Book of All Forbidden Arts, Heresy, and Sorcery). Kindle edition. First published 1475.

Hatsis, Thomas. 2015. *The Witches' Ointment: The Secret History of Psychedelic Magic.* Rochester, Vt.: Inner Traditions/Bear & Company.

Hayes, Antoinette N., and Steven G. Gilbert. 2009. "Historical Milestones and Discoveries That Shaped the Toxicology Sciences." *EXS* 99: 1–35.

Heiser, Charles B. Jr. 1969. *Nightshades: The Paradoxical Plants.* San Francisco: WH Freeman.

Hesse, O. 1901. "Über die Alkaloïde der Mandragorawurzel." *Journal für Praktishe Chemie* 64: 274–86.

Hildegard von Bingen. 1998. *Hildegard von Bingen's Physica: The Complete English Translation of Her Classic Work on Health and Healing.* Translated by Priscilla Throop. Rochester, Vt.: Healing Arts Press.

Holzman, Robert S. 1998. "The Legacy of Atropos, the Fate Who Cut the Thread of Life." *Anesthesiology: The Journal of American Society of Anesthesiologists* 89, no. 1: 241–49.

Hurwitz, Siegmund. 2009. *Lilith—The First Eve: Historical and Psychological Aspects of the Dark Feminine.* Translated by Gela Jacobson. Einsiedeln, Switzerland: Daimon-Verlag.

Huson, Paul. 1972. *Mastering Witchcraft.* New York: Penguin/Corgi Childrens.

Jackson, Betty P., and Michael I. Berry. 1979. "*Mandragora*—Taxonomy and Chemistry of the European Species." Chap. 39 in *The Biology and Taxonomy of the Solanaceae,* edited by J. G. Hawkes, R. N. Lest, and A. D. Skelding, 505–12. London: Academic Press.

Jackson, Nigel. 1996. *Masks of Misrule.* Taunton, UK: Capall Bann.

Juvin, Phillippe, and Jean-Marie Desmonts. 2000. "The Ancestors of Inhalational Anesthesia: Soporific Sponges (XIth–XVIIth Centuries); How a Universally Recommended Medical Technique Was Abruptly Discarded." *Anesthesiology* 93: 265–69.

Kaldera, Raven. 2011. *Northern Tradition Shamanism: The Shamanic Herbal.* Hubbardston, Mass.: Asphodel Press.

Laguna, Andrés. 1554. *Annotations on Dioscorides of Anazarbus*. Lyon, France: Guillaume Rouillé.

Lee, M. R. 1999. "The Snowdrop (*Galanthus nivalis*): From Odysseus to Alzheimer." *Journal of the Royal College of Physicians of Edinburgh* 29, no. 4.

———. 2006. "The Solanaceae II: The Mandrake (*Mandragora officinarum*): In League with the Devil." *Journal of the Royal College of Physicians of Edinburgh* 36: 278–85.

———. 2007. "The Solanaceae IV: Atropa belladonna, Deadly Nightshade." *Journal of the Royal College of Physicians of Edinburgh* 37, no. 1: 77–84.

Lewin, Louis. 1998. *Phantastica: A Classic Survey on the Use and Abuse of Mind-Altering Plants*. Rochester, Vt.: Park Street Press. First published 1929.

Maestas, Silence (Jessica). 2007. *The Little Red Man: Fly Agaric in History and Culture*. Hubbardston, Mass.: Asphodel Press.

Martin, Deborah J. 2013. *Baneful! 95 of the World's Worst Herbs*. Sparks, Nev.: Herb Lady.

Mathers, S. Liddell MacGregor, trans. and ed. 2000. *The Key of Solomon the King* (Clavicula Salomonis). Foreword by R. A. Gilbert. Boston/York Beach, Maine: Weiser Books. First published 1889.

Mayor, Adrienne. 2009. *The Poison King: The Life and Legend of Mithradates, Rome's Deadliest Enemy*. Princeton, N.J.: Princeton University Press.

Meyer, Joseph E. 1934. *The Herbalist*. Hammond: Indiana Botanic Gardens.

Middleton, J. Henry. 1892. *Illuminated Manuscripts in Classical and Mediaeval Times*. Cambridge, UK: University Press.

Miller, Richard. 1983. *The Magical and Ritual Use of Herbs*. Rochester, Vt.: Destiny Books.

———. 1985. *The Magical and Ritual Use of Aphrodisiacs*. Rochester, Vt.: Destiny Books.

Müller-Ebeling, Claudia, Christian Rätsch, and Wolf-Dieter Storl. 2003. *Witchcraft Medicine: Healing Arts, Shamanic Practices, and Forbidden Plants*. Translated by Annabel Lee. Rochester, Vt.: Inner Traditions.

Pendell, Dale. 2010. *Pharmako Gnosis: Plant Teachers and the Poison Path*. Berkeley, Calif.: North Atlantic Books.

Pennick, Nigel. 2005. *Practical Magic in the Northern Tradition*. Leicestershire, UK: Thoth.

Plaitakis, A., and R. C. Duvoisin. 1983. "Homer's Moly Identified as *Galanthus nivalis* L: Physiologic Antidote to Stramonium Poisoning." *Clinical Neuropharmacology* 6: 1–5.

Porta, Giambattista della. 1558. *Magiae Naturalis, sive, De Miraculis Rerum Naturalium* (Natural Magic or The Miracles of Natural Things). Naples, Italy: Matthias Cancer.

Rätsch, Christian. 2005. *The Encyclopedia of Psychoactive Plants: Ethnopharmacology and Its Applications.* Foreword by Albert Hofmann. Rochester, Vt.: Park Street Press. First published 1998.

Rätsch, Christian, and Claudia Müller-Ebeling. 2013. *The Encyclopedia of Aphrodisiacs: Psychoactive Substances Used for Sexual Practices.* Rochester, Vt.: Park Street Press.

Remington, Joseph P., Horatio C. Woods et al. 1918. *The Dispensatory of the United States of America.* Twentieth edition. Philadelphia: Lippincott.

Retief, Francois P., and Louise Cilliers. 2019. "Poison, Poisonings, and Poisoners in Rome." Chap. 15 in *Toxicology in Antiquity,* edited by Philip Wexler, 231–42. London: Academic Press.

Rosarium, Catamara, Jenn Zahrt, and Marcus McCoy. 2015. *Verdant Gnosis.* Revelore Press.

Roth, Harold. 2017. *The Witching Herbs: 13 Essential Herbs and Plants for Your Magical Garden.* Newburyport, Mass.: Weiser Books.

Ruck, Carl A. P., Jeremy Bigwood, Danny Staples, Jonathan Ott, and R. Gordon Wasson. 1979. "Entheogens." *Journal of Psychedelic Drugs* 11, no. 1–2: 145–46.

Schulke, Daniel A. 2012. *Veneficium: Magic, Witchcraft and the Poison Path.* Rancho Boca de la Cañada del Pinole, Calif.: Three Hands Press.

———. 2017. *Thirteen Pathways of Occult Herbalism.* Rancho Boca de la Cañada del Pinole, Calif.: Three Hands Press.

Schultes, Richard Evans. 1976. *Hallucinogenic Plants.* Houston, Tex.: Golden Press.

Schultes, Richard Evans, Albert Hofmann, and Christian Rätsch. 1992. *Plants of the Gods: Their Sacred, Healing, and Hallucinogenic Powers.* Rev. ed. Rochester, Vt.: Healing Arts Press. First published 1979.

Scot, Reginald. 1886. *The Discoverie of Witchcraft.* London: Elliot Stock. First published 1584.

Siegel, Ronald K. 1989. *Intoxication: Life in Pursuit of Artificial Paradise.* New York: E. P. Dutton.

Simoons, Frederick J. 1998. *Plants of Life, Plants of Death.* Madison: University of Wisconsin Press.

Stedman, T. L. 1942. *Stedman's Shorters Medical Dictionary. Poisons and Antidotes.* Westchester, Ill.: Wilcox & Follet.

Stewart, Amy. 2009. *Wicked Plants: The Weed That Killed Lincoln's Mother and Other Botanical Atrocities*. Chapel Hill, N.C.: Algonquin Books.

Thomas, H., and M. Wentzel. 1898. "Über mandragorin." *Chemische Berichte* 31: 2031–37.

Thompson, C. J. S. 1968. *The Mystic Mandrake*. New York: University Books.

Tu, Tieyao, Sergei Volis, Michael O. Dillon, Hang Sun, and Jun Wen. 2010. "Dispersals of Hyoscyameae and Mandragoreae (Solanaceae) from the New World to Eurasia in Early Miocene and Their Biogeographic Diversification within Eurasia." *Molecular Phylogenics and Evolution* 57, no. 3: 1226–37.

Tupper, Kenneth W. 2009. "Entheogens and Existential Intelligence: The Use of Plant Teachers as Cognitive Tools." *Canadian Journal of Education* 27: 499–516.

Ungricht, Stephan, Sandra Knapp, and John R. Press. 1998. "A Revision of the Genus Mandragora (Solanaceae)." *Bulletin of the Natural History Museum, Botany Series* 28, no. 1: 17–40.

Voogelbreinder, Snu. 2009. *Garden of Eden: The Shamanic Use of Psychoactive Flora and Fauna, and the Study of Consciousness*. Australia: Self-published.

Yuruktumen, A., S. Karaduman, F. Beni, and J. Fowler. 2008. "Syrian Rue Tea: A Recipe for Disaster." *Clinical Toxicology* (Philadelphia) 46, no. 8: 749–52.

ONLINE RESOURCES

Cech, Richo. 2019. "Growing Mandrake—Beyond the Basics." *Richo's Blog*. Strictly Medicinal Seeds website.

Church, Stephen, and Carol Church. 2009. "Harvesting & Making Specific Tinctures." The Herbarium website.

Cleversley, Keith. 2002. "Artemisia vulgaris—Mugwort." Entheology.com.

———. 2002. "Atropa belladonna—Belladonna." Entheology.com.

Gillabel, Dirk. 1988. "Nigredo—Blackness," "The Peacock's Tail," "Albedo—Whiteness," and "Rubedo—Redness." Chaps. 1.3–1.6 in *Alchemical Concepts* (online book). Soul-guidance.com website.

Hunter, M. Kelley. 2017. "Lilith in Astrology: The Meaning of the Black Moon Lilith in Astrology." Astrology Club website.

Jaana. *Herbal Picnic* blog.

Marina. "The Three Liliths." Dark Star Astrology website.

McCoy, Daniel. Norse Mythology for Smart People. Norse-mythology.org.

McIntyre, Anne. Fellow of the National Institute of Medical Herbalists and Member of the Ayurvedic Practitioners Association. Annemcintyre.com.

Northern Tradition Paganism. Northernpaganism.org.

Oates, Shani, and Robin the Dart. People of Goda, Clan of Tubal Cain website.

Index

Page numbers in *italics* indicate illustrations.